JUICE

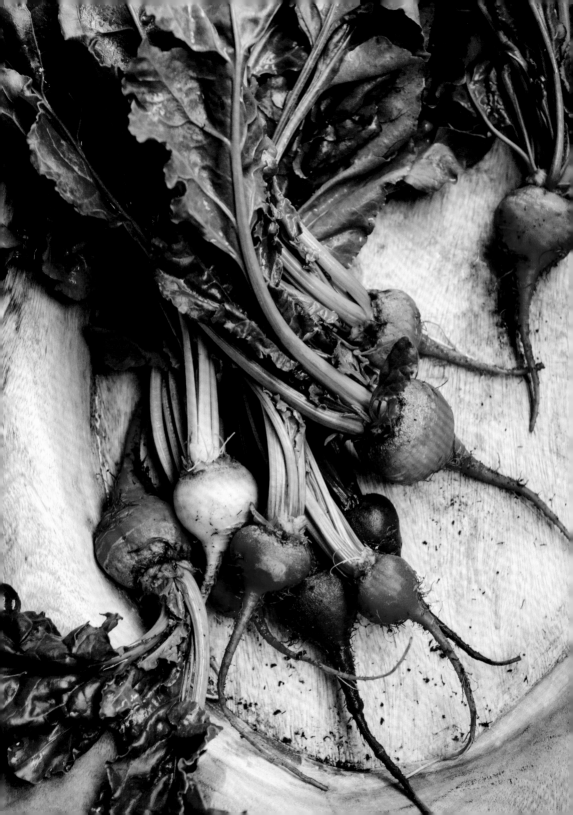

JUICE

RECIPES FOR
JUICING, CLEANSING
& LIVING WELL

Carly de Castro, Hedi Gores & Hayden Slater
FOUNDERS OF PRESSED JUICERY

Photography by Anaïs & Dax

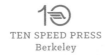

TEN SPEED PRESS
Berkeley

Drink Your Fruits
and Vegetables

JUICING 7

The Juice Box

RECIPES 37

Push Reset

CLEANSING 109

ACKNOWLEDGMENTS

First and foremost, a huge thank-you to our incredible contributors. This list includes, but is not limited to, Dr. Alejandro Junger, Natalia Rose, Shelley Young, Kris Carr, Daphne Oz, Dr. Harold Lancer, and Pamela Salzman. Each of you has inspired us at some point in our lives to be conscious of what we put into our bodies and rethink what it means to live a healthy life. We are honored that you have shared some of your wisdom on these pages.

To Sandra Bark, what can we say? We could not have done this without you. This is a project that is so close to our hearts, and you handled it with such love and care. We feel incredibly grateful that you were willing to take the plunge with us, making sense of our thoughts and finding words where we didn't think we had any. More than anything, you gave us confidence in our knowledge and ability to tell this story. It's been such a fun process, so *thank you*!

To Justin Camilo, we can taste the love in every juice you make, and your guidance during this process has been invaluable. Thank you for believing in this journey and sticking with us every step of the way—and for teaching us that kale can, in fact, taste like candy.

To Amanda Baker, Eugene Kim, and Suzanne Hall, thank you for always being willing to step in and advise us during this process. And to our entire Pressed Juicery team, we are so grateful for the community effort that goes into every project at this company.

To Lauren Felts, our favorite nutritionist, thanks for all of your hard work in getting us what we needed, even on tight deadlines, and for checking our research and not being afraid to edit.

To Julie Bennett, Katy Brown, and everyone at Ten Speed Press, thank you for asking us to write this book. Working with you has been a wonderful experience, and it has been an honor to be published by a team that we respect so much. We appreciate your willingness to let us be ourselves and stay true to our voice and our mission.

To Anaïs and Dax, Vivian Lui, and Scott Horne, what a fun and wonderful experience we had shooting with you. Watching you bring our recipes to life with each of your unique talents was such an honor.

To our agent, Erin Malone, you believed in this book from the moment we met you. Thanks for standing in our corner and looking out for us. It has been a true pleasure.

To Becka Oliver, thanks for being willing to give advice to a few novice writers, and for helping us assemble a stellar team.

To our families and friends, an endless thank you for the support and laughter throughout this entire ride. Especially to Alisa, Kate, and David, for getting your hands dirty and recipe testing late into the night, and to Alejandro, for your love and advice, always. And to Gavin and Luca, thank you for challenging us every day to reach higher and be better. We love you.

Most importantly, to our customers and readers, you are the core of Pressed Juicery and the reason we come to work every day. We would be nowhere without your support and dedication to living well. Thanks for letting us be a part of your journeys. You inspire us.

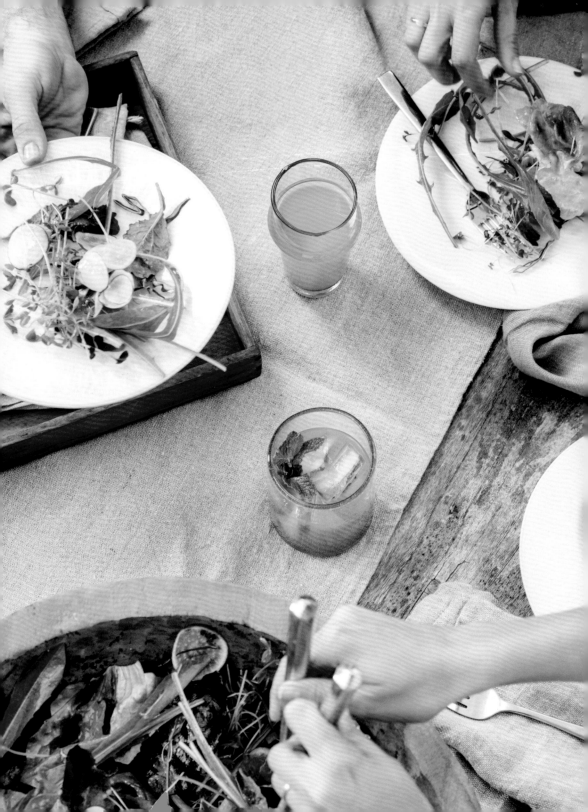

SHARING THE JUICE,
or Why a Successful Juice Company Would Give Away All of Its Recipes

BY CARLY DE CASTRO

What do you do when you wake up in the morning? How do you energize, uplift, and get yourself going? We all have our little rituals, the things that we do to feel bright eyed and ready for the day ahead. For all of us at Pressed Juicery, drinking a green juice in the morning is one of our rituals, like washing our faces or brushing our teeth. It's something we do every day, without even thinking about it. We do it because we know how good it makes us feel—because it gives us a lift, replenishes our nutrient levels, and tastes amazing. When we're on the road and fresh juice isn't within easy access, we miss our juice. We're so grateful when we are home or at the shop and can easily drink a glass brimming with green goodness. Juicing has become more than a habit for us; it's a priority and one of the ways that we care for ourselves.

Our devotion to juice is the origin story of Pressed Juicery, and it is the reason for this book: because at Pressed, we think the real secret to a healthy and happy life shouldn't be a secret at all. The proof is in these pages. Everything we've learned over the past decade on our juicing journey is here for you to share.

Whether your goal is to add a glass of green juice to your daily routine or take the plunge and see what cleansing is all about, this book is your invitation to experience the impact that drinking fresh fruit and vegetable juices each day can have on your mind, body, and soul so you can move through your day at full capacity instead of feeling sluggish or as if you're operating in a mental fog. What we hear from customers all the time is that health and vibrancy are much sought-after states of being—everybody wants to feel amazing and alive! But too many people are missing the mark on how to achieve these states. Balance is hard to come by these days, or so it seems. But it is not impossible! Juicing is a simple and powerful way to support your health and the health of your family.

From choosing the right style of juicer to learning the difference between juicing and blending, discovering how to pick produce, and making delicious juices, this book has everything you need to know to bring the juice home. We call it our cookbook/how-to juice guide/cleansing manual/produce handbook. In short, it's an all-around guide to making juices at home that will completely wow your taste buds. We've got sweet juices and savory juices, spicy juices and creamy nut milks, and smoothies and refreshing flavored waters and elixirs. Your body needs quality nutrients! Why fall into the trap of fast and convenient food and beverage options when you can have fast, convenient servings of fresh, delicious juice? When it comes to juicing, once you start making the effort, it stops feeling like work—or rather, the work feels worth it. Give it a try and you'll see what we're talking about!

how a green juice changed my life

The amazing effect that juicing can have on your life and your whole being is something that I have experienced personally. When I was in my early twenties, before I discovered juicing, my main form of vegetables was the iceberg lettuce on my hamburger. Whatever I felt like eating, I ate. Meanwhile, I felt sluggish and out of shape, depressed and unmotivated, and I wondered constantly why I felt so *low*.

I was twenty-two when I hit 175 pounds, and that's when I decided I'd had enough. I had tried various fad diets, and none of them worked. I needed to make a change—not just in my diet, but also in the way that I lived my life.

I began reaching out to friends and family, asking for advice. One friend advised trying green juice. So I began buying a fresh green juice at my local market on the way to work. It completely energized me. It was different than the diet sodas and sugary juices I was used to; I felt remarkable. I hadn't felt that

GREENS, ROOTS, AND CITRUS

In this book, you'll discover that the foundation of the Pressed Juicery menu, our style of cleansing, and many of our recipes involve these elements:

GREENS—juices based on leafy green vegetables

ROOTS—our most filling juices, based on root vegetables like beets and carrots

CITRUS—our light, delicious, immune boosters

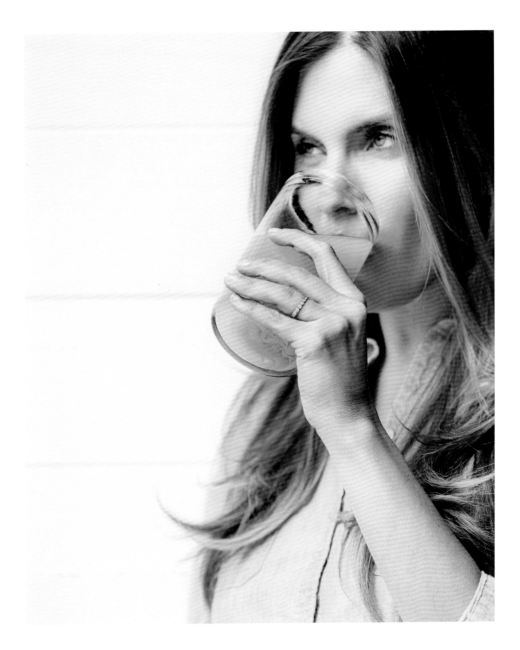

SHARING THE JUICE

energetic since I was a child, and my moods noticeably improved.

So I began reading books about raw food and juicing. Over the next year or so, I began making my own juices at home and experimenting with various ingredients. I slowly stopped craving unhealthy foods and started reaching for fruit in place of cookies, and salads in place of pizza. There was no coach breathing down my neck or forcing me to do this—my body was telling me what it needed and what it craved, and for the first time, I felt empowered.

On my journey, I ended up losing about forty-five pounds and gaining a new life and a new perspective. And it all began with drinking green juice every day.

To me, this was pretty powerful stuff. I had spent so much time buying into the idea that it was complicated to be healthy and fit, that once I figured out the magic set of rules to follow, I would become an ideal version of myself. Instead, I learned that there are many options for living a healthy life. The shift that I required was to develop a new perspective on what healthy *means* to find out how I fit into the puzzle.

the pressed juicery story

Pressed Juicery is really a passion project that began with a conversation between friends. After the way my health had turned around, I had been thinking about how I could do something with my life that would incorporate what I had learned so I could share it. So I called my friend Hayden Slater to tell him

what was on my mind. "You're not going to believe me, Carly," he said, "but Hedi and I are talking about exactly the same thing right this minute."

It turned out that Hayden and our mutual friend Hedi Gores had been having a cup of tea and talking about creating a healthy food or beverage concept that could make people's lives better. Same thing at the same time? I don't believe in coincidences. . . .

When the three of us sat down together to talk it over, what emerged from our conversation was the realization that we had all changed our lives through juicing. We had learned that cleansing our bodies and getting rid of the toxins with juice was an effective way to get to the root of what our bodies were telling us they needed: drinking juice, eating alkaline foods, getting a healthy dose of physical exercise, and steering clear of negative energy in any form. What we all found on our own paths was that the real key to feeling our best and looking our best was *balance*. Because when we drank our green juice, we felt clean, and we were able to find that balance more readily.

We wanted to tell everyone what we had discovered: *juice!* We had taken different roads, but our personal journeys had led us to this place and this moment, when we had a revelation; we were three people with a single, clear idea.

Pressed Juicery was born out of the belief that in order to find fulfillment and balance each day, modern people need to be armed with a fresh set of tools that are simple, convenient, and tailored to their hectic schedules. We believe that everyone is entitled to live their best lives, but for this to happen, we need vital nutrients so we can function at our optimal levels.

Juicing provides a convenient way to meet those requirements. With the founding of Pressed Juicery, we gave the people juice. Now, we want to teach you *how* to juice.

So, if you are **interested in juicing but have not yet tried it** . . .

You will learn the basics about what juicing does for you and instructions on how to make juices at home.

If you are **battling health issues** . . .

You will find numerous recipes and facts about how juicing and cleaning up the way you eat can improve the state of your health

If you are **an experienced "health nut"**. . .

You will learn facts about the history of cleansing that you may not have known and discover how to reboot your system. You'll also find detailed information on body alkalinity as well as recipes to add to your repertoire.

If you are **dealing with a weight problem** . . .

You will gain tools and insight into what may be causing your weight gain and how to manage it with healthy eating tips and recipes.

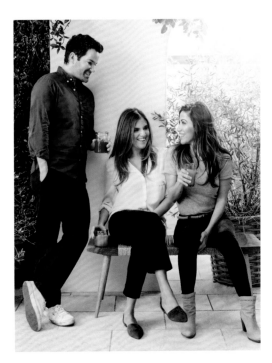

We believe that juice is a way for people to *get back to their roots*. To do this, we start simple, with fruits and vegetables, the most nourishing and natural foods we can possibly put into our bodies. We aim to cut through the confusion and bring people simple and delicious opportunities to be better and live better every day. We wrote this book for the same reason we started Pressed: because juicing is a life changer. It changed our lives. What can it do for you?

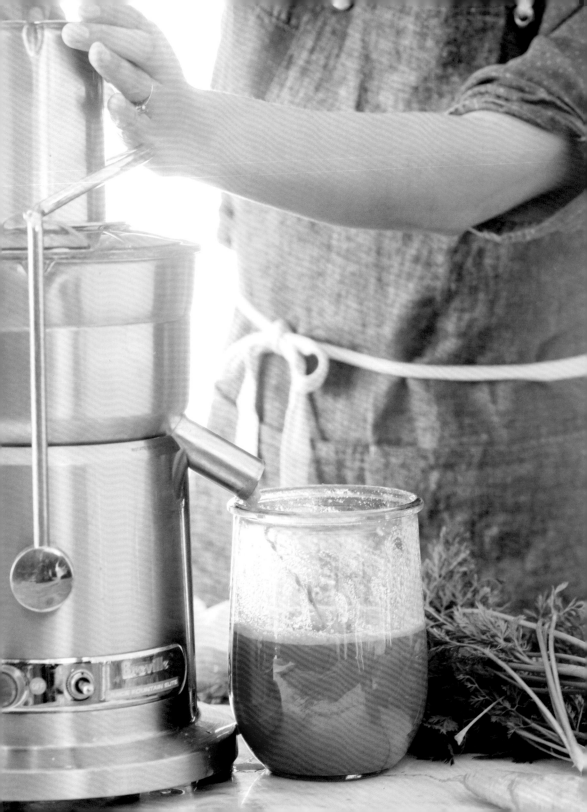

DRINK YOUR FRUITS
AND VEGETABLES

JUICING

If you've ever visited one of our shops or been to our website, you know that our mantra is *Get back to your roots*. We believe that in order to find fulfillment and balance each day, we need ways to incorporate health into our lives that are convenient instead of stressful and as common as a morning coffee but packed with nutrients and vital energy. We believe that for everyone to live their best lives, we need to get back to our roots: back to the fruits and vegetables that give us health. All you need is a juicer and a blender, and you'll have your daily juice whenever you want it, however you want it.

If you want to fall in love with fruits and vegetables, or you already love them and want to enjoy them in new and delicious ways; if you crave new flavors and want to tantalize your taste buds on a daily basis; if you're bored of "from concentrate" supermarket offerings; if you want to put the spring back in your step and the glow back in your skin, and give yourself all the nutrients your body craves, join us.

Because a glass of juice a day can really add up to something amazing.

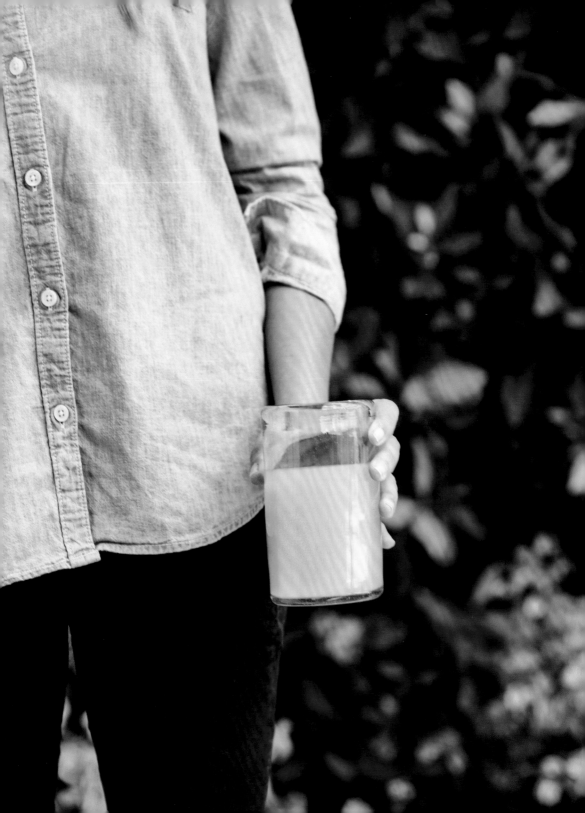

CHAPTER 1

HERE'S TO YOUR HEALTH

Our juice is one part of the everyday, healthy ways that we at Pressed Juicery live our lives. How will juice fit into your life? Everybody does it differently. Some people drink a green juice instead of a morning coffee because it provides clean energy to start the day. Other people drink fresh juice instead of having a handful of potato chips as their afternoon snack. Still others take it to another level and spend one day, or three days, or, for more experienced juicers, five or more days, solely drinking juice as a form of cleansing.

Our foundational belief is that any regimen by which you add healthful juice to your diet, along with fresh fruits and vegetables and whole grains, is about getting clean. Juicing is always about getting clean: putting the healthy stuff in, flushing the toxins out, and keeping the pathways clear and the goodness going. When people cleanse, solid foods are replaced with juices for a few days so the digestive system can reset and regain equilibrium. If you've already juiced, you

know what we're talking about. If you haven't cleansed yet, remember, just getting the green stuff in is an amazing first step toward taking care of your health! (If you're interested in cleansing, you can learn all about it in the cleansing section; see page 109.)

Because that's part of why you're here, isn't it? If you're anything like our customers, your health is something that you think about a lot. You want to stay healthy, you want to get healthier, but sometimes it just seems overwhelming. So many of our customers walk through our doors with the misconception that achieving health and wellness has to be a complicated ordeal! And it's no surprise that people are confused. Most of what we are told by doctors and scientists in mainstream media implies that health is a quantifiable puzzle that needs to be solved. Every other day, a new piece of information or a study surfaces that tells us that some new pill or surgery will be able to fix our problems and lead to better health.

At Pressed, we see health as a holistic process in which your daily choices and habits have a profound effect on your state of well-being. Ideally, what you consume every day not only feeds your body but also actually makes you *feel* and *look* your best. We believe that when you change the framework and look at it from a different perspective, your understanding of what it means to be healthy changes in a powerful way.

We are not doctors. We are not scientists. We are human beings who have experienced the powerful energy surge that comes from putting more natural vitamins and minerals into our systems. Good nutrition equals a healthier state of being. Our habits define us, and once we move away from habits that don't serve us and incorporate habits that are good for us, well, everything begins to change.

Modern medicine provides us with a vast amount of knowledge and information that helps keep us well, but we believe that being healthy is about more than going to the doctor and getting your shots. The World Health Organization defines health as the absence of disease. But we want to be more than just *not sick*. We want to be thriving. Energetic. Feeling as though we could leap tall buildings in a single bound.

Going to the doctor for a regular checkup and when you don't feel well are important parts of taking care of yourself—but they are *not* the same thing as truly taking care of yourself on a daily basis. When it comes to your health, you get what you give. So if you want to get healthy, get energized, and feel amazing, you must give yourself the best stuff on earth.

We are talking about fruits and vegetables.

JUICING VERSUS BLENDING

You could never eat as much raw produce (or consume as much in a smoothie) as you can incorporate in a juice. While blending is a great form of consuming fruits and veggies, juicing is a more direct way to get nutrients without having to run the full plants through the digestive tract. That said, smoothies make you feel fuller longer and can be a fantastic meal replacement; they just serve a different purpose than juices do.

Personally, we love incorporating both juices and smoothies into our regimens—and we have provided an array of our very favorite smoothie recipes (see chapter 8) for you to experiment with. We don't believe in rules when it comes to eating (or drinking!) for health— if it's good for you, throw it in and see if you like the taste. There are plenty of wonderful ingredients—like avocados, bananas, and dates—that cannot easily be juiced and are perfect as a base for a blended drink.

For advice on buying a blender, see page 89.

why juice?

It will probably not surprise you to hear us say that fresh produce is an essential factor for good health. We've all been told to eat our fruits and vegetables since we were kids, and most of us were probably not so sure how we felt about that green mass quivering on the side of the plate. Most people know that consuming a diet rich in unprocessed foods, whole grains, and primarily composed of fruits and veggies is good for us and will keep us strong and healthy. But if we know that, why aren't we all healthier?

Think about your own daily dosage of fruit and vegetables: Are most of the fruits and vegetables that you eat cooked or raw? If the answer is "cooked," consider that cooking produce causes it to undergo chemical and enzymatic changes. These changes make it less likely that we will get all of the potential nutrients out of a given item of food, because so many of these nutrients have been killed by the application of heat.

If your answer is "raw" and you are thinking to yourself that you eat a lot of raw vegetables, think about how much "a lot" is. Eating salads on a regular basis is fantastic, of course, but how much do you really eat? You'd need to eat about 5 pounds of kale, spinach, romaine, cucumber, celery, and parsley just to get the nutrition you get in one glass of our green juice!

While you may understand that fresh, nutritious food is good for you, and you may often choose salads and soups and stir-fries over burgers and mac and cheese, it's possible that you're not getting the high levels of nutrients and enzymes present in the fruits and vegetables you eat. And if you're not getting all the good stuff, how can you truly benefit from their incredible potency? Often, even just having to digest large quantities of produce makes it less likely that you will really benefit from the full nutritional value of what you are consuming.

This is where juicing comes in.

Juicing allows for the nutritional wonders that are fruits and vegetables to be easily and efficiently absorbed by the body. And it increases the nutritional quotient. It would be very challenging to eat as many vegetables in one sitting as you can easily drink in juice form—think about how full you would be and the extra load on your digestive system!

The main purpose of the digestive system is to break down food to extract the water and nutrients and to get rid of the fiber. Juicing reduces your system's workload and takes care of that first step by breaking down the food for your body. Drinking juice is an easy, delicious way to get your nutrients—and you feel the results quickly and powerfully. We think of it as our daily dose of medicine— pure liquid nourishment that rebuilds our cells from the inside out, boosts the immune system, and simply makes us feel amazing.

A WORD ON JUICING

BY ALEJANDRO JUNGER, MD

After Dr. Alejandro Junger graduated from medical school in Uruguay in 1990, he moved to New York City to work at New York University and then Lenox Hill. Moving to New York lead to a drastic change in his lifestyle and diet, which soon showed up as irritable bowel syndrome and depression. The realities of what it was like to be a patient of the system in which he practiced was such a shock that he began to search for an alternative solution to his health problems. His findings are the subject of his first book, Clean, a manual for readers who want to learn how to turn on and work their own detoxification systems to restore and maintain optimal health.

It is thought that our ancestors started cooking around two million years ago. This was a huge discovery! Once cooking was invented, it allowed our brains to grow bigger because our bodies needed to spend less time digesting massive amounts of food. Cooking changed things forever. It changed us.

Juicing is huge and almost as important an invention as cooking. Juicing allows us to condense vitamins and minerals without having to eat massive amounts of produce. And even better, it also allows us to condense the nutrients without losing them to heat. This preserves all the great things our bodies need to boost immunity, improve energy, and be less susceptible to disease.

Think of your body as the hardware of your computer and the food you eat as the software. The software tells your body how to run and which good genes to turn on and bad genes to turn off. When you focus on upgrading the quality of the food you eat, you in turn upgrade the quality of the information you send to your body. As a result, your body runs better on a daily basis and becomes less susceptible to disease in the long run.

You have to think of juicing like we think of cooking! Just as the invention of cooking did all those years ago, juicing is also changing humanity, and I highly recommend incorporating it into your whole-foods diet.

what's in your juice?

Most of us don't really think about what actually makes up fresh juice—it's just fruits and veggies, right? Look a little closer, and within that gorgeous glass of green, orange, or red is a nutritious mix of water, protein, carbohydrates, amino acids, vitamins, and minerals that are essential to good health.

WATER

Your fruits and vegetables contain a high percentage of water, so it makes sense that most of that water is released into the fresh juice that you drink. We all know we need to drink more water—our bodies consist of between 50 and 65 percent water, and our systems depend on water for survival because it flushes out toxins from our organs and delivers nutrients to our cells. Lack of water, or dehydration, can lead to some serious issues, such as compromised cardiovascular function and renal impairment. We find that juicing gives us a running start when it comes to the 2 to 3 quarts of water per day that we are supposed to be drinking. Drinking juice is an incredible way to stay hydrated—you get many of the benefits of drinking water, but you also get many more nutrients from the fruits and veggies you are consuming. Win-win!

PROTEIN

Yes, fruits and vegetables have protein, too. You might not think of fruits and vegetables as a prime source of protein, but when they are juiced, their nutritional qualities become concentrated, making them an excellent source of easily absorbed amino acids (the building blocks of protein). Nut milks are a great protein source, too.

CARBOHYDRATES

Carbohydrates are a main energy source for the human body and the backbone of your nutritional profile. Before they are juiced, fruits and vegetables are sources of both simple carbohydrates (sugars) and complex carbohydrates (including fiber), which are not the same as the refined carbohydrates found in food items like cookies and brownies. Compared to vegetable juice, fruit juice contains more sugars. We find that it's best to consume more veggies than fruit for this reason.

FATS AND OILS

Our bodies need essential fatty acids to thrive, and lucky for us, although most fruits and vegetables have low levels of fat, they do contain trace amounts of some of the essential fatty acids that our bodies need, like linoleic acid, which help our bodies produce energy. Then there are the fruits and vegetables like avocados and coconuts that are high in healthy fats, unusual in the fruit and vegetable kingdom and very lucky for us, because they are delicious additions to juices that pack a big nutritional punch. If you are juicing and would like to add more healthy fats to your routine, try a juice blended with avocado, coconut meat, or chia seeds (see the smoothies in chapter 8).

VITAMINS AND MINERALS

Vitamins and minerals like iron, calcium, and vitamin C are crucial for your health, but your body can't produce them, so you must get them from your food. Eating citrus fruits, greens, and root vegetables gives us vitamins A, B, C, D, E, and K. It also gives us magnesium, selenium, potassium, phosphorus, and a host of other micronutrients. All of these help to keep your brain functioning, your eyes seeing, and your body producing red blood cells to build and repair your muscles, and so on.

what's not in your juice?

A question we often get from customers is "What happens to the fiber in juice? Isn't fiber a *good* thing?" Yes! Fiber is great, and surprisingly, juicing actually does provide some fiber, particularly soluble fiber, which has been shown to lower cholesterol levels.

One of the major purposes of cleansing is to let your digestive system rest by giving it a break from fiber. However, drinking your fruits and veggies on a regular basis in the form of juice should be in addition to, not instead of, the raw and cooked vegetables you eat with your meals. These vegetables give you an extra dose of nutrients along with all the fiber you need. And as you start making juice at home, you'll notice that the fiber from the fruits and vegetables is left over as pulp, which can be used in baked goods and other recipes to add fiber, as well as in skin treatments and baths. And there's another thing that isn't in your juice: all of the processed, acidic foods that eventually build up in your system, leading to symptoms of chronic disease and illness.

the alkaline trip

Your body's pH balance is one of the pillars on which your good health rests. Your pH reflects how acid or alkaline your system is, and that relates to the foods you eat. Did you know that every food and substance we put into the body leaves an ash residue after the body metabolizes it? This residue is either alkaline or acidic, depending on the mineral composition of the foods and the way we digest them.

In order for your vital organs to function properly, your body requires an alkaline environment. Enjoying alkaline fruits and vegetables in the form of fresh, raw juice instead of relying on acidic foods—which include foods that have been canned, frozen, or cooked—makes your body more alkaline, helping bring balance to your system and life.

At the other end of the spectrum are high-acid foods that produce excess acid waste, which is a cause of inflammation and, many

HEALTH BENEFITS OF SOLUBLE FIBER

Juice *does* contain soluble fiber. Here's why we love it.

- Lowers blood cholesterol levels and helps to normalize blood glucose and insulin levels

- Reduces blood pressure

- Reduces risk of certain forms of cancer, including colon cancer

- Benefits gastrointestinal health

- Enhances weight control

CONCENTRATE ON THIS

What's the difference between fresh-pressed juice and the stuff you find on grocery store shelves? Check the labels for the following terms: *concentrate*, *made from concentrate*, and *not from concentrate*.

- Concentrate: This means the water content has mostly been removed, making it easily transportable.

- Made from concentrate: This means it is made from concentrated juice with water added back in.

- Not from concentrate: This means it is fresh juice that has been bottled and shipped, and it has usually been heat-pasteurized.

The important thing to remember is that most of the enzymes and nutrients are killed in the heat-pasteurization process, while fresh-pressed juice delivers all of the enzymes and nutrients. When reading any juice label, you always want to look for the words *100 percent juice* and make sure there are no additives or preservatives.

---

believe, the root of disease. If your diet is high in meat, cheese, white flour, white sugar, and processed food, or if you drink alcohol or smoke cigarettes, then it is possible that you are suffering from ailments such as acne, joint pain, premenstrual syndrome, asthma, depression, flus and colds, migraines, food allergies, heartburn, low energy, low libido, insomnia—the list goes on and on. Advanced symptoms of overacidity include cancer, Crohn's disease, schizophrenia, and multiple sclerosis.

Alkaline-forming foods are the only answer to combating overacidity. So which foods are alkaline forming and which foods aren't?

- **Extremely alkaline:** Foods that are extremely alkaline forming taste fresh; they include fruits and veggies of all kinds and herbs and spices such as ginger, parsley, and cayenne.

- **Moderately alkaline:** Sprouted grains, olive oil, and soy products are moderately alkaline.

- **Neutral:** Raw cow's milk, cream, and butter are all neutral (but they have to be raw).

- **Slightly acidic:** Any food that is cooked, canned, or frozen is slightly more acidic than it would be otherwise. The same goes for any chemically grown, processed food.

- **Very acidic:** And then there are the extremely acidic products, like meat, cigarettes, drugs, and carbonated drinks.

Since fruits and vegetables are all alkaline, adding juice to your diet adds alkalinity, which creates a physical environment of wellness and health. And another plus: Drinking fresh juice on a regular basis can make you start craving foods that live on the alkaline side of the street. In the long run, this can add up to big positive changes in your health. Tailoring your diet to mostly alkaline-forming, fresh foods—for example, every single recipe in this book—might just be the shift that changes everything for you.

how to go alkaline

The easiest way to increase alkalinity in your body is to eat more fresh, plant-based foods and limit your consumption of toxins. Many of the most alkaline foods are also used to heal illnesses (ginger, lemon, honey), so it makes sense that ingesting them as a preventative measure might prove to be quite effective.

A WORD ON DRINKING GREEN
BY NATALIA ROSE

Natalia Rose is one of our favorite experts on detox, raw food, and healthy living. She is the author of many books that were transformative tools during our journeys to health, including The Raw Food Detox Diet.

Raw green vegetable juice is one of the key "nonnegotiables" in the health protocols I design for my clients. When we juice leafy greens like kale, spinach, chard, and even romaine lettuce, we receive the greatest blood cleanser available to us—pure, alkaline, and rich with chlorophyll! Juicing enables us to take in epic amounts of this chlorophyll-infused substance, what I call the life force, because once the mechanism of juicing separates the fiber from the liquid (which I think

of as the blood of the plant), we can take in a lot more liquid than we possibly could if it was still connected to the fiber, because it would be too much bulk. Contrary to popular belief, excessive fiber is not beneficial! When you are eating one or two raw vegetable salads a day, it is unnecessary to stock up on extra fiber.

In my search for the most healing substance in the world, nothing compares to raw, organic, fresh-pressed greens. This juice instantly infuses the body (like a blood transfusion) with chlorophyll and countless vitamins, minerals, and enzymes. Nothing could be a more effective detoxifying tool. And it's refreshing and delicious!

If you want to go alkaline, there are a few things that you can focus on: what and how you eat and how you feel emotionally. Alkaline foods, eaten in the right ratio, combined properly, and chewed well, will result in an alkalized body. So will exercise, soothing and relaxing environments, meditation, and love! (Sounds pretty good, doesn't it?)

- Start each day by drinking 1 cup of warm water mixed with 1 teaspoon lemon juice, 1 teaspoon manuka honey (which is highly alkaline and incredibly healing), and 1 tablespoon apple cider vinegar. We call this our Morning Alkalizer (page 138).

- Drink green juice, which is one of the most alkalizing beverages you can consume.

- Maintain a diet with an 80 to 20 percent ratio of alkaline-forming foods to acid-forming foods.

- Combine your foods appropriately: eat your starches with vegetables and your protein with vegetables, and don't mix meat and potatoes.

- Make exercise and meditation regular parts of your day.

To achieve an optimal immune system, glowing skin, better mood, and weight loss, join us on our alkaline trip. It starts with green juice and extends to all areas of your life, because after all, health is about feeling great inside and out. To really get the full benefits of your juice, we encourage you to care about what you put in your mouth at mealtimes and also about the lifestyle that gives your meals context. How do you behave during mealtime? Are you relaxed and appreciative or rushed and stressed? Being flexible and open and getting plenty of rest, laughter, fresh air, love, and physical activity, along with healthy foods and juices, are all ways to maximize alkalinity and keep stress and inflammation at a minimum.

Just opening this book is a step toward a more balanced, vibrant, and happy you. Now you understand why it is so important to add juice to your diet, eat and drink alkaline foods, and avoid processed, acidic foods. What amazing benefits will you get from your green juice? An alkalized, energized body; a new connection to your health; and a revitalized understanding of how what you drink and eat influences how sharp or cloudy your mind is. But first, you need a juicer.

A WORD ON ALKALINITY

BY SHELLEY YOUNG

Shelley Young and her husband, Dr. Robert Young, are the vital forces behind The pH Miracle book series, alkalizing supplements, and therapies. Their powerful philosophy on keeping an alkaline diet and lifestyle, what Dr. Young calls the New Biology, has been a breakthrough concept in health and nutrition since the early 2000s. The Youngs have guided thousands in their pursuit of health and healing with an alkaline diet.

Just as the earth has an external environment that has to be kept clean and clear for fresh air and pure water, each of us has an internal environment that must also be kept clean and clear. Like internal rivers and streams, our veins, arteries, and lymphatic vessels must run pure for optimal health and strength.

Making fresh green juice a part of my daily diet, along with eating alkaline foods, has afforded me the great blessing of superb health. At age sixty, I am still able to run strong, wear the same size I did in high school, and am pain- and drug-free.

In a nutshell, I am pH balanced thanks to the chlorophyll-rich diet I eat and the healthy way I live. Many people who travel to my pH Miracle Ranch from all over the world come here to learn how to get pH balanced themselves. They lose their aches and pains, their skin becomes more youthful, and they return to their ideal weight. It's miraculous! All from making our food our medicine, and our medicine our food! Hippocrates—and Popeye—were right! Eat (juice) your veggies!

To stay balanced, I suggest that you eat and drink at least 80 percent high-water-content, chlorophyll-rich foods and beverages and 20 percent mildly acidic foods and beverages. If you can manage 90 to 100 percent alkalinizing foods and drinks, even better. Fresh green juices are ideal for this!

ALKALINE-ACID FOOD CHART

ALKALINE FOODS Stick to salads, fresh vegetables, and healthy nuts and oils. Try to consume plenty of raw foods and at least 2 to 3 quarts of clean, pure water daily.

ACID FOODS Steer clear of fatty meats, dairy, cheese, sweets, chocolates, alcohol, and tobacco. Packaged foods are often full of hidden offenders, and microwaveable meals are full of sugars and salts. Overcooking also removes all of the nutrition from a meal.

VEGETABLES

Artichoke	Comfrey	Onion
Arugula	Coriander	Parsley
Asparagus	Cucumber	Peas
Basil	Endive	Pumpkin
Beet	Garlic	Radish
Bell pepper	Ginger	Red cabbage
Broccoli	Grasses	Rhubarb
Brussels sprouts	Green beans	Rutabaga
Cabbage	Kale	Spinach
Carrot	Kohlrabi	Sprouts
Cauliflower	Leek	Squash
Celery	Lettuce	Turnip
Chives	Mustard greens	Watercress
Collard greens	New potato	Zucchini
	Okra	

FRUITS / FATS & OILS

FRUITS	FATS & OILS
Avocado	Borage
Coconut	Evening primrose
Grapefruit	Flax
Lemon	Hemp
Lime	Oil blends
Pomegranate	Olive oil
Tomato	

SEEDS, NUTS & GRAINS

Almonds	Caraway seeds	Lentils
Any sprouted seeds	Cumin seeds	Sesame seeds
Buckwheat groats	Fennel seeds	Spelt
	Hemp seeds	

OTHERS

Hummus

Sprouts (soy, alfalfa, mung bean, wheat, radish, chickpea, broccoli, etc.)

Tahini

MEATS

Beef	Seafood (apart from occasional oily fish such as salmon)
Chicken	
Lamb	
Pork	Turkey

FRUITS / DAIRY

FRUITS	DAIRY	
All fruits, aside from those listed in the alkaline column.	Cheese	Milk
	Cream	Yogurt
	Ice cream	

CONVENIENCE FOODS

Canned foods	Instant meals	Powdered soups
Chocolate	Microwaveable meals	
Fast food		Sweets

DRINKS

Beer	Coffee	Fruit juice
Carbonated/ fizzy drinks	Dairy smoothies	Spirits
		Tea

FATS & OILS / SEEDS & NUTS

FATS & OILS		SEEDS & NUTS
Corn oil	Saturated fats	Cashews
Hydrogenated oils	Sunflower oil	Peanuts
Margarine (worse than butter)	Vegetable oil	Pistachios

OTHERS

Artificial sweeteners	Soy sauce
Biscuits	Tamari
Condiments (tomato sauce, mayonnaise, etc.)	Vinegar
	White bread
Eggs	White pasta
Honey	Whole wheat bread

Source: www.phmiracleliving.com/t-food-chart.aspx

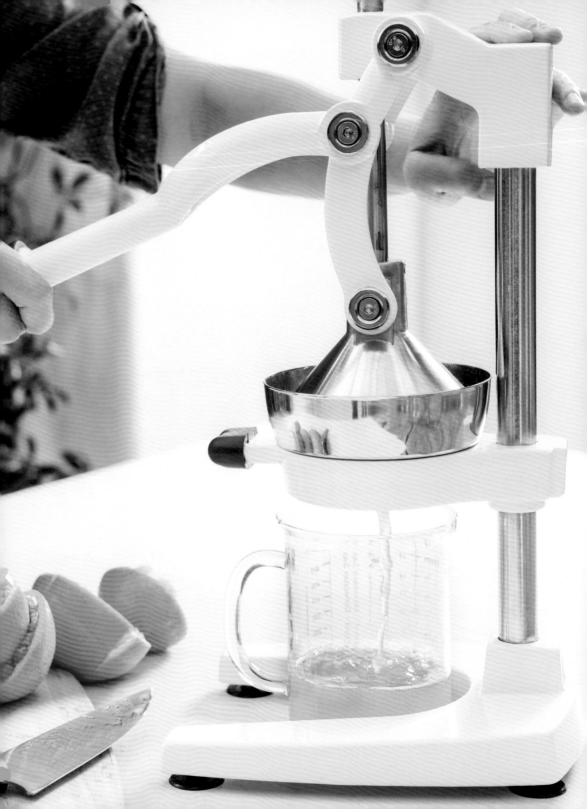

CHAPTER 2

THE BASICS OF JUICING

An incredible glass of juice begins with the right equipment and some gorgeous, organic ingredients. That's what we're going to talk about in this chapter. We'll start with equipment, covering everything you need to know about juicers, from the different types to their machinery, value, and price points. Next, we'll explain how blenders and juicers can work together to support your health and your juicing. Finally, we'll dish about all of the incredible fruits, vegetables, and herbs that we love to use and show you the best ways to store and prepare your produce. We'll also introduce you to an array of superfoods that you can use to boost your juice. Even if you've never so much as squeezed an orange, you can learn how to create drinks that will delight and impress. So fill your fruit bowl, pack your pantry, and enjoy a completely personalized menu of fresh, delicious juices in the comfort of your own kitchen.

choosing the best juicer for you

There are a number of methods by which juice can be extracted from fruits and vegetables: from masticating juicers that "chew" produce to more classic styles that work by shredding and pressing. All juicers have benefits, so please consider your personal priorities. Some juicers will save you money, others will save you time, and still others will produce juice that has a longer-than-normal shelf life. And some juicers are desirable just because they are quieter than the others. So do some research before you buy. This guide to our favorite juicers showcases best features, concerns, and noise ratings.

THE CHEWERS: MASTICATING/SLOW JUICERS

This type of juicer has one slow-turning gear, or auger (a fancy word for a drill bit), that masticates the produce; that basically means that it chews it. This breaks down the fiber and cell walls to form pulp. The machine then squeezes the pulp to extract the juice, which contains a high level of nutrients, enzymes, and trace minerals.

PROS:

· Extracts more juice than a centrifugal juicer.

· Operates at a slow speed, minimizing heat and oxidization.

· Juice retains most of its nutrients.

· Juice can be stored for up to 48 hours in the fridge.

CONS:

· Expensive, will run $200 to $300.

· Juice contains more fiber and pulp.

THE CLASSICS: CENTRIFUGAL JUICERS

One of the oldest types of juicers around and the most popular home juicer, the centrifugal juicer uses a grater, or shredder disk, and a strainer basket to hold the pulp. The produce is put in the top of the machine, and the disk shreds the fruits and veggies at high speeds while the juice is released into a spout.

PROS:

· A lot of produce can be loaded in at one time.

· Juices can be made quickly.

· Affordable, decent models start at $75.

CONS:

· Short shelf life: spinning and heat causes oxidization, so you need to consume the juice very quickly.

· Pulp builds up relatively quickly inside the juicer and must be dumped out to make room for more.

· Not as effective with leafy vegetables. Usually a good deal of pulp is left wet, meaning that there is juice left in the pulp that must be discarded.

THE DOWNLOAD ON DECIBELS

If you're the type to sleep with earplugs, the noise factor of your juicer may be something to consider. The higher the speed at which a juicer operates, the more noise it will produce. The twin-gear juicer and the hydraulic press are less noisy than the centrifugal juicer, and the masticating juicer is somewhere in between.

Generally speaking, juicing is not the quietest of activities. We like to imagine that the sound of the motor is revving us up; it's actually quite a fun way to start the day, and we try to enjoy it.

THE TWINS:
TWIN-GEAR/TRITURATING JUICERS

These juicers have two interlocking gears and work at low speeds to slowly press fruits and veggies. The produce is shredded and then squeezed between the gears until the pulp is nearly dry and almost all of the juice is squeezed out.

PROS:

- Juice retains most of its nutrients.

- The low speed results in less oxidization and less nutrient destruction from heat.

- Juice lasts up to 72 hours stored in the fridge.

- Produces very dry pulp, which means that it maximizes the amount of liquid yielded from the produce.

CONS:

- It takes longer than a centrifugal juicer to extract juice.

- Cleanup can be time-consuming.

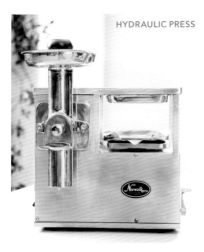

HYDRAULIC PRESS

THE FERRARIS:
HYDRAULIC PRESS JUICERS

A hydraulic press is perhaps the finest of juicers. It works through a two-part process: produce is first fed through a shaft where a rotating grinder disk shreds it into a very fine pulp. The pulp is released into a mesh bag, and then the filled bag is placed on a hydraulic press tray and a lever is pulled to activate the press. At this point, pressure (a *lot* of it) is applied to press the bag and extract basically every bit of juice—and the nutrients, enzymes, minerals, and phytonutrients that come with it! No air touches the juice during this process, so it spoils less easily. This is the type of juicer that we use at Pressed Juicery. We realize that a hydraulic press is not a realistic choice for many because it can be very expensive and because it is a time-consuming process.

PROS:

- Produces no oxidization or foam.

- Extracts 100 percent more juice than a centrifugal juicer and 50 percent more juice than a masticating juicer.

- Pulp is completely dry and often color-free, which means the nutrient-dense pigmentation goes straight into the juice.

- Juice lasts for 72 hours stored in the fridge, so you have to make juice only every couple of days.

CONS:

- Expensive, will run upwards of $1,000.

- Time-consuming process. Give yourself at least 15 to 20 minutes to make a batch of juice.

stocking your juice pantry

Now that you've set up your juicing equipment, it's time to experiment with all the fantastic ingredients you can run through it. We believe that juicing should be playful and fun. We've included heaps of recipes in this book, but we'd also like to invite you to take the basics you learn here and go wild! How? Stock your refrigerator with all of the luscious produce you can find, and then pack your pantry with our juicing flavor boosters.

Juicing at home is a very personal thing. Some people prefer a sweet juice (add apples and beets), while others like it light and lemony (add cucumbers or citrus) or tangy and spicy (add lemon or ginger). The combinations are endless, and it's really up to you and your taste buds to decide what you like. Obviously, you will be juicing fruits and vegetables most often, so let's start there.

FRUITS

We're all familiar with fruit juice. Who didn't grow up drinking a tall glass of OJ with breakfast (poured from a container or made from frozen concentrate) or slurping an apple juice box at the park or quenching a hot summer day with lemonade (which is essentially lemon juice and sugar). All three of these fruits—oranges, apples, and lemons—are star ingredients in many of our recipes. We have used them in what we hope will be new and interesting ways that go way beyond the ordinary. You'll see that when made fresh, apple juice has a delicately sweet flavor that is fantastic as a base for vegetable juices. A squeeze of tart lemon can be a wonderful balance for a combination of that sweet apple and sharper leafy greens. You want OJ with your breakfast? Sure. How about combining it with lettuce, cilantro, and pineapple for a tropical twist? And then there are so many other fruits—from berries to melon, grapes, kiwi, and more—that we put to work in our recipes, all of them with their own unique flavors and benefits. As we will continue to tell you, there are no rules to combining flavors, only a willingness to get your hands a little stained and taste test. The possibilities are endless.

As a rule of thumb, we like to lightly peel all citrus fruits to keep the flavor relatively mild, but if you prefer the rind, it won't hurt you to juice it. We do, however, remove the rind of any fruit whose rind is simply too hard to juice, such as pineapple and melon. For fruits with softer, milder-tasting skin, as well as fruits with pits, we tend to throw it all in. As you gain comfort and confidence as a juicer, have fun experimenting and create your own set of rules.

VEGETABLES

As you're about to find out, we are a little obsessed with veggies around here. From greens to roots to savory juices, we use vegetables in some creative and unusual ways, and we are excited for you to expand your palate and to taste foods in liquid form that you've had only in side dishes. Vegetables come in all shapes and sizes, and many of them have leaves and skin that might leave you a bit confused. In general, we like to leave the skin on most vegetables, from carrots to beets. But there are certain veggies, like cucumbers, which have particularly

THE DIRTY DOZEN

When you're juicing or eating raw fruits and veggies in salads, it's great to eat organic if you can afford it and it's available. Most of us don't have the budgets to go organic all the time, so here's a way to simplify: remember that some fruits and vegetables have higher pesticide residues than others. That means that nonorganic varieties of those particular edibles—called the dirty dozen (plus kale and collard greens and summer squash)—are the ones you want to keep out of your juice and out of your home. Keep this list handy and prioritize your choices to make the healthiest decisions you can without cramping your wallet or your style.

The next time you go to the market, look for organic for the following fruits and veggies:

Apples	Cucumbers	Nectarines (imported)	Spinach
Bell peppers	Grapes		Strawberries
Celery	Hot peppers	Peaches	Summer squash
Cherry tomatoes	Kale and collard greens	Potatoes	

If you're buying commercial fruits and vegetables, just make sure to wash them extra carefully (see page 39).

bitter-tasting skin, that can alter the flavor of your juice (and not in a good way). We prefer to peel cucumbers, unless you happen to use Persian or English cucumbers, whose skin is milder. We also peel ginger before juicing it because we prefer the flavor of ginger without the bitter peel.

For leafy greens—that's romaine, spinach, kale, chard, collards, dandelion greens, and the like—we simply wash them and run them through the juicer, including stems, which contain vitamins and minerals that you don't want to miss out on.

Vegetables such as fennel, carrots, and beets have long stems with leaves. We like to use the leaves (or fronds) from time to time, but usually we cut off the stems. It's up to you to try out the flavors and see for yourself what you prefer.

In general, depending on what juicer you have, you will need to coarsely chop your fruits and veggies in order to make them fit into the mouth of the machine. You can do this however you like, and it will not affect the flavor of your juice.

STORING YOUR PRODUCE

If you've spent any time perusing the produce section of the grocery store, you have probably noticed that some of the fruits and veggies are kept in coolers, while others are on display in the center of the room. Here is an easy guide to help you remember which ones need to be kept in the fridge (this is really important!), which ones should be left to ripen at room temperature, and those that can go either way.

With the exception of onions, garlic, and potatoes, most vegetables need to be refrigerated. Fruits are a different story, however. Some must ripen before they are picked while others can be left to ripen after picking. For the ones that still need to ripen, it is best to leave them at room temperature. The chart below will help you store your fruits properly to get the best flavor and the longest shelf life.

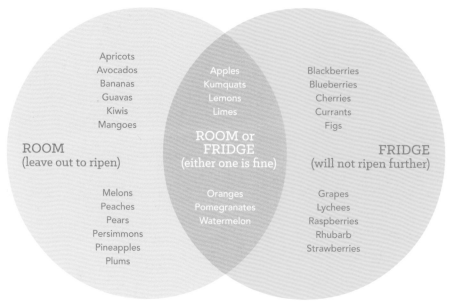

ROOM VERSUS REFRIGERATOR:
WHICH FRUITS RIPEN AFTER BEING PICKED?

Apricots
Avocados
Bananas
Guavas
Kiwis
Mangoes

Apples
Kumquats
Lemons
Limes

Blackberries
Blueberries
Cherries
Currants
Figs

ROOM
(leave out to ripen)

ROOM or
FRIDGE
(either one is fine)

FRIDGE
(will not ripen further)

Melons
Peaches
Pears
Persimmons
Pineapples
Plums

Oranges
Pomegranates
Watermelon

Grapes
Lychees
Raspberries
Rhubarb
Strawberries

HERBS

While most of us know them as flavor enhancers that spruce up a roast or a salad, herbs like parsley, mint, cilantro, basil, and dill have a number of excellent nutritional qualities that, along with their strong flavors, make them a fantastic addition to juices and smoothies. As you read through the recipes, you'll learn all about these benefits—and as you use them in your juices, you'll come to appreciate their distinctive and invigorating flavors. We use herbs in our recipes liberally—often a small handful—and find that they can really set the tone for the taste of a drink. All you really have to do is wash them well and toss them in, keeping the stems on unless otherwise noted. As far as flavor combinations, mint tends to give juices an uplifting zing, while parsley and basil add more of an earthy, savory tone. Play around with them and see what you think!

JUICE BOOSTS

By following the recipes in this book, you'll be using heaps of kale, spinach, arugula, apples, and lemons to create the foundation of your juices. To this we add what we call a juice boost, our favorite feel-good and flavor enhancers, which make the finished juice extra delicious and super healthy. Home cooks have arsenals of spices and condiments that improve the flavors of their meals; juicers also have their secret weapons. Our suggestions are below. Have fun, try something new, or kick things up a notch. (Our recommendations for the brands we love are in the Resources, page 144.) For additional inspiration, flip to the elixir recipes starting on page 103, which feature many of these ingredients and superfoods.

ALOE VERA Aloe vera is known for its ability to heal the intestinal lining, which is key for a healthy digestive system. It moves through the intestinal tract absorbing toxins, which are then carried through the colon and eventually eliminated. People with stomach issues such as bloating, constipation, and ulcers would benefit from the regular use of aloe vera. It is also loaded with antibacterial properties, reduces inflammation, and is great for the skin. Aloe is truly one of our favorite ingredients! Use the gel version topically on the skin like a moisturizer, and add the liquid version to juices or purified water as a drinkable delight. We highly recommend using a couple of tablespoons of aloe vera as a boost on a daily basis and especially during cleansing.

APPLE CIDER VINEGAR The benefits of apple cider vinegar are practically limitless: for generations, it has been a go-to remedy for curing everything from indigestion to allergies and the flu. It may not have the most delicate aroma, but don't let its sharp olfactory presence deter you from incorporating this incredible tonic into your life. We can't emphasize enough just how much we endorse apple cider vinegar for its ability to alkalize the body and improve digestion by increasing hydrochloric acid in the stomach.

We've already discussed how important it is to maintain an alkaline system (see page 14), and this ingredient really packs a punch in that area.

A WORD ON RADIANT SKIN

BY DR. HAROLD LANCER

Hedi says, "I've known Dr. Lancer for years, and I'm always telling friends just how amazing he is. I love how he's always on the forefront of skin care breakthroughs—and how committed he is to drinking juice and using natural ingredients. We all want skin that glows with radiance and health, and that is precisely Dr. Lancer's expertise." At his Beverly Hills–based dermatology practice, he follows a less-is-more approach when developing bespoke skin care treatments for his patients. People come from around the world for Dr. Lancer's care because the results are simply remarkable.

Diet has a noticeable and lasting impact on your skin. Eating healthily is an essential part of keeping skin looking young, while eating processed food and simple carbs is detrimental to sustaining a youthful appearance. In junk food, all of the natural nutrients are replaced by synthetic additives. When you shift to eating and drinking whole and raw foods, you learn how to taste real flavors again, you are taking care of your body, and you will look younger.

Raw fruits and vegetables are great for your skin. Consider the following:

- Processed foods lose living enzymes and nutrients, including vitamins, minerals, and fiber.

- Nutritional deficiencies show on your skin.

- Raw fruits and vegetables contain more water and add hydration to the body; hydration means healthy skin.

Juicing is an easy and efficient way to consume exponentially more fruits and vegetables than one would in an average meal. The vitamins, minerals, and antioxidants provided by juicing contribute to long-term overall health—and glowing and radiant skin. When you juice, you can customize, matching your unique taste preferences while you deliver these vital nutrients to your entire body.

Want more radiant, youthful looking skin? Try adding pomegranates and kiwis to your juices. Pomegranates have a unique compound called punicalagin, a powerful antioxidant, and high levels of vitamins A, C, and K. Pomegranate's antioxidant properties protect skin from free radical damage, which has both anticancer and antiaging benefits. Vitamin K has been shown to increase the elasticity of the epidermis and speed healing for wounds. These healing and regenerative properties are excellent for your skin. Kiwis are a great source of vitamin C and vitamin E, both of which are essential vitamins for your skin. Vitamin C promotes the production of collagen, which is necessary for reversing visible signs of aging, such as fine lines and wrinkles. Adding both of these ingredients to your juice will be especially beneficial for skin care.

BEE POLLEN Bee pollen is the substance that collects on the legs of honeybees as they travel from flower to flower and gets brought back to the hive to feed the young bees. Possibly *the* quintessential superfood, bee pollen is incredibly nutrient dense. It is believed to contain more than a dozen vitamins and minerals and more than five thousand enzymes, in addition to a range of amino acids and fatty acids. It's no wonder that bee pollen is appreciated for its abilities to improve immunity and make the body feel good.

While many people think that honey in its natural form contains bee pollen, it actually doesn't. So when you take bee pollen as a supplement, you are getting vitamins and minerals that aren't available in other bee products.

CACAO NIBS OR POWDER Chocolate that's good for you? Yup. That's what we're saying! In its natural form, raw cacao is rich with antioxidants—higher than blueberries and even the superfoods acai and goji berries! According to health experts, raw cacao is a great source of magnesium and iron, as well as the feel-good chemicals phenylethylamine and anandamide, which make us feel alert and happy. We use cacao anytime we want to get a chocolaty flavor in one of our drinks. Blend up some fresh mint, coconut meat, and cacao, and you have a mint chip shake. Freeze it and voilà—healthy mint chip "ice cream"!

CELTIC SEA SALT Many people shy away from using salt because of its high sodium content, but our bodies actually *need* salt to survive. Most of the table salt that you find these days is stripped of its nutritional value. Adding good-quality sea salt to your diet is a whole other story. Unrefined, mineral-rich sea salt provides a percentage of magnesium and other trace elements that are essential to health, and it has the added benefit of being free of other potentially toxic agents that are added to table salt, such as anticlumping and flowing agents, aluminum, and even chlorine, which is used for bleaching. We use Celtic sea salt—our favorite type—as an ingredient in our almond milk, which also helps mellow out the sweet flavor.

SKIN SUPERFOODS

Promote healthy, glowing skin by drinking your daily fill of the following:

Aloe vera	Kiwi
Apple	Lemon
Chlorophyll	Mint
Cucumber	Parsley
Ginger	Pomegranate
Kale	Spinach

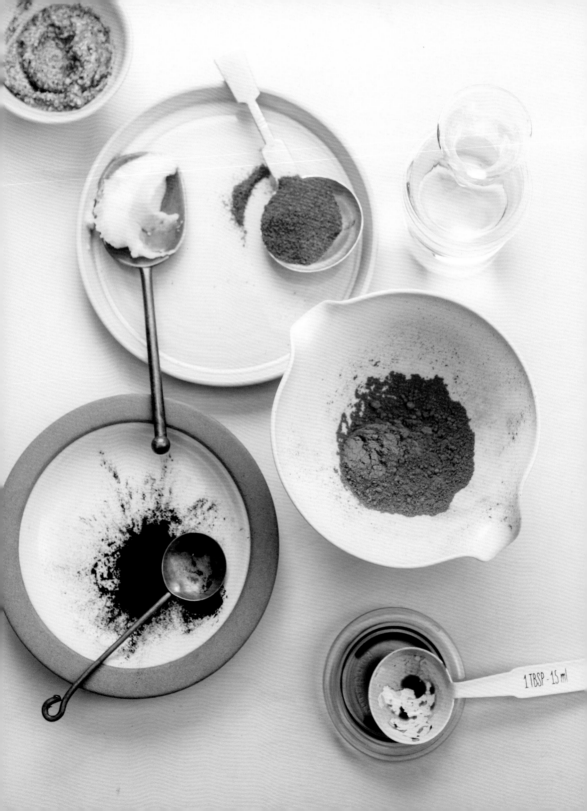

CHIA SEEDS Chia is a powerful little super-food from Central and South America that was a staple of the Mayan people's diet and has recently gained popularity. Chia seeds contain about 11 grams of fiber per ounce; they are also one of the richest sources of omega-3 and omega-6 fatty acids and contain disease-fighting antioxidants. (You may have noticed that we're big on antioxidants around here.) In addition, the seeds have twice the protein of any other seed or grain and *five* times the calcium of milk.

One of the great things about chia seeds is that you don't need to eat many of them to get their benefits: just 1 tablespoon at a time will give your health a big boost. And when you add chia seeds to a liquid, they expand to nine times their volume, taking on the consistency of a pudding. Some people love the gelatinous texture, while others are confused by it, but don't let the unfamiliar texture put you off. Just like aloe, chia's consistency is what makes it a powerful lubricant and bulking agent, which keeps your colon happy and your bowels moving along.

CHLOROPHYLL You probably remember chlorophyll from your high school science classes—it's the pigment that turns plants green. This idea is actually really amazing. If the green veggies we eat are the lifeblood of a healthy diet, and chlorophyll is the lifeblood of the veggies themselves, then chlorophyll is the purest form of green vegetables and a powerful health booster. (It's so meta!)

Let's go back to those science classes for a minute: Chlorophyll is vital for photosynthesis—the process by which plants absorb energy. As a plant "breathes," the chlorophyll in the plant absorbs sunlight, carbon dioxide, and water and converts them via a chemical process into energy that the plant can use. This transformed energy is basically made up of sugar and oxygen; the sugar feeds the plant and helps it grow, while the oxygen is released into the atmosphere as waste—and then inhaled by the rest of us for our survival. It's a pretty fantastic relationship. Chlorophyll also supplies magnesium and antioxidants, which is why it has a reputation for preventing disease.

You get the basic idea—this stuff is great for our health. You get a dose of chlorophyll in any fruits and veggies you consume, but we love it so much that we're all about adding a liquid supplement to our water or juice. As dosage varies, please check the information listed on your supplement.

CINNAMON This delicious, warming spice goes great with apples, pumpkins, and autumn—and has been helpful in reducing blood sugar and cholesterol levels, in addition to boosting metabolism. Studies show that consuming just ¼ teaspoon of cinnamon a day may reduce blood sugar levels, which has sparked a conversation about its use for treating type 2 diabetes. And just like other spicy foods, cinnamon boosts metabolism and has been found to aid in weight loss.

COCONUT OIL Coconut oil is getting a lot of love right now. Known for containing healthy saturated fats, coconuts are rich in antimicrobial and antifungal properties, and the oil can be used for sautéing veggies, topically treating skin disorders, and boosting metabolism and thyroid function. It's great for high-heat cooking, too. Because coconut oil can tolerate high temperatures, cooking with it is a lot healthier than less stable oils, which break down the hotter the pan gets.

For our purposes, we like to ingest coconut oil raw: 1 to 2 tablespoons added into smoothies and juices, with a little left over to moisturize our hands.

E3LIVE E3Live is one of the most magical supplements we've ever taken. It is the world's only frozen, organic, blue-green algae, wild harvested from Klamath Lake in Oregon. It is filled with more than sixty-five vitamins, minerals, amino acids, and essential fatty acids that support the immune system and promote physical and mental health in a variety of incredible ways. It is the highest known source of natural vegetable protein (58 percent) in the world, making it a great choice for vegans. You can purchase E3Live online, and while it is on the pricier side, you can literally feel it working immediately through your system.

FLAXSEED OIL Packed with high levels of alpha-linolenic acid, flaxseed oil (linseed oil) provides high levels of omega-3 essential fatty acids. It has become well-known for its ability to aid in hormone balance as well. You can take flaxseed oil by the spoonful, but if that doesn't work for you, just add it to a juice and you'll barely know it's there. One thing to be careful of is spoilage. Flaxseed oil tends to get rancid easily, so buy it in a dark-colored bottle, keep it refrigerated, and never heat it. Add a spoonful to salads, juices, smoothies, and grain or vegetable dishes after cooking.

GINGER Ginger is crucial to your diet, which is why we use it in so many of our juices. You have probably eaten spicy pickled ginger as a complement to a sushi dinner, but have you ever consumed it in pure liquid form? If not, it's a must-try. Ginger contains anti-inflammatory compounds called gingerols, which have been known to reduce joint pain and generally boost the immune system. A member of the same plant family as turmeric—another amazing immune booster—ginger has long been used as a treatment for intestinal problems from nausea to gas. If your mother ever gave you ginger ale for a stomachache, think along those same lines, minus the sugar and preservatives.

Ginger has also been used in Eastern medicine to heat the body, which improves circulation, and to boost the metabolism, which aids in weight loss.

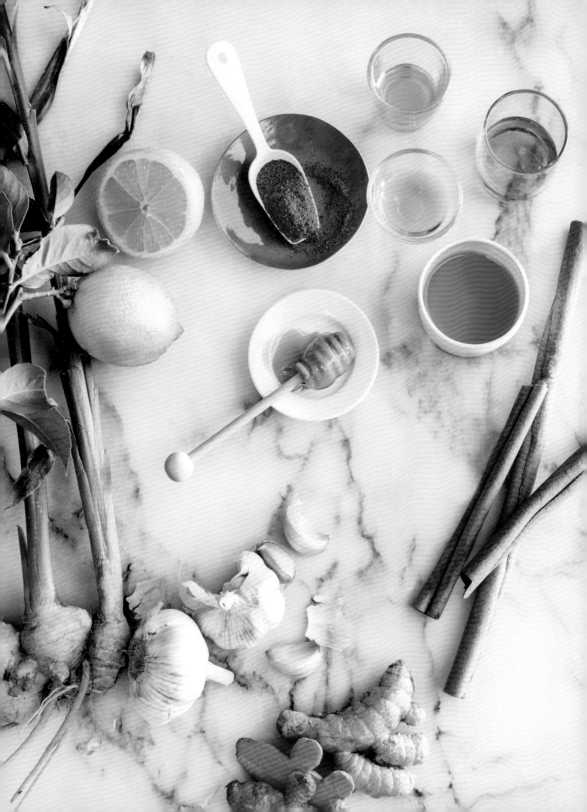

MACA POWDER An Incan superfood, maca powder is a renowned adaptogen, having the ability to promote balance in the body, especially in the endocrine system. Maca helps the body cope with stress, both physical and mental. In addition, it can balance your hormones and generally improve energy, and we all need that! Add a scoop to your smoothie in the morning to energize in a natural way.

MANUKA HONEY A rose is a rose is a rose, but all honey is not created equal. There are as many different kinds of honey as there are flowers, and all honeys are directly influenced by the climate in which the bees live and the plants in proximity to their hive.

The methods of harvesting and processing the honey once it leaves the hive are the steps we are most concerned with. Most store-bought honey is heated (and some brands are even cut with corn syrup), which kills off the beneficial compounds and leaves just its sugary taste. Raw unprocessed honey, on the other hand, contains antioxidants, minerals, amino acids, enzymes, and all sorts of other potent components. It's a true superfood and one with healing properties so great that it has been used for centuries to treat internal and external wounds (think sore throats and skin problems).

All raw honey naturally contains health benefits and can be used to boost the immune system and treat certain ailments. But when we want a little extra boost, we choose manuka honey. This is the Rolls-Royce of honey. Manuka honey is produced solely in New Zealand by bees that pollinate the manuka bush. Manuka honey is known for

its active potency as a therapeutic substance used to treat inflammation and heal wounds. It is the only honey in the world that has been tested for its healing abilities and is a natural antibiotic. Manuka honey is labeled with a rating, which denotes how potent each jar is. Anything above a ten is considered medicinal grade. Use it as you would any other honey—a teaspoon or two to taste.

OLIVE OIL It's pretty likely that you already have olive oil in your pantry, but this incredible natural lubricant deserves to be recognized as more than something we use to sauté our side dishes and dress our salads. Olive oil contains monounsaturated fatty acids (MUFAs), which are the same healthy fats found in avocados and certain nuts. MUFAs are known for their ability to help lower cholesterol levels and protect our cells from damage.

Have a spoonful in your smoothie, or even straight, before bed a couple of nights a week. No joke; it gets things moving in the colon. And be sure to buy high-quality, extra-virgin olive oil that has been packaged in a dark-colored bottle. Because oils are easily destroyed by light and heat, it's important to store your olive oil in a cool, dark place. Otherwise, the oil can become rancid, which degrades not only its flavor, but also its nutrient profile.

OREGANO OIL Widely recognized as a treatment for a variety of infections and diseases, oregano has anti-infective properties, and when the oil is extracted in its purest form, it is a potent weapon against illness. Oregano oil contains more than fifty compounds that

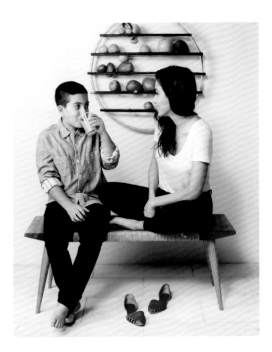

It has been widely tested for its health benefits and even some Western doctors have endorsed it as part of a healthy diet. The active compounds in turmeric, known as curcuminoids, are potent phytonutrients that contain powerful antioxidant properties. It is a blood cleanser as well and promotes liver and kidney detoxification. While many people consume turmeric in capsule form or as a culinary spice, we like to add it to juices or water for a direct boost to our immune systems.

The first juice we ever made came from a recipe. It's incredible that a list of ingredients has the power to shift the course of somebody's life, like a magic potion. How will you choose the first juice you make? Will it be based on your favorite fruit? Will it be an at-home version of one of your favorite juices from our stores? Is there a boost that caught your eye while you were reading through the list above?

So ladies and gentlemen, get ready to start your juicers. Because in just a few pages, you will have the power to make green juices, fruit juices, smoothies, nut milks, elixirs, and more. All you need is a pantry full of inspiration and the willingness to try something new.

support the immune system, and it contains protective antioxidants as well. When you ingest oregano oil, you can feel it working almost immediately. Look for wild Mediterranean versions and take it straight (according to the instructions on the bottle) if you feel a cold coming on. But be careful: it's spicy. You can also take it with other liquids, such as water or juice.

TURMERIC This incredible root is an anti-inflammatory superfood that also acts as an antibacterial and antiseptic in the body. Turmeric is in the same family as ginger, and the fresh root looks like a small, orange ginger root. It has been used for centuries as part of Ayurvedic medicine in India. Turmeric is most notable for its anti-inflammatory properties, which have the potential to fight diseases such as cancer, arthritis, heart disease, and stomach conditions.

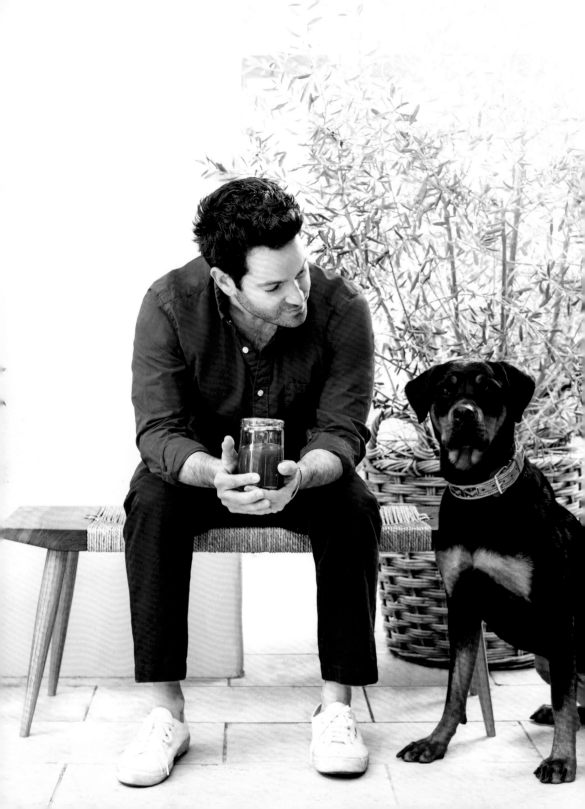

THE JUICE BOX

RECIPES

At Pressed Juicery, we focus on three categories of juices as the basis for our menu, our cleanses, and now our book. But that's just the beginning. There are *so* many ways to drink your fruits and veggies. The following chapters show you how.

It's All about the Greens: Kale, spinach, romaine, collards . . . our green juices are made up of mostly leafy green vegetables, and we've come up with some unique recipes that really pack a punch in terms of flavor. These are the foundation for our cleansing program and give you an easy and delicious way to get your daily dose of veggies in liquid form.

Get Back to Your Roots: Beets and carrots . . . these are nutritionally dense vegetables that taste great, too. Our flavor combinations appeal to all different taste buds and utilize some interesting ingredients with amazing health benefits. We consider our roots juices to be our most filling juices.

Citrus Appeal: Grapefruit, orange, lemon . . . our customers love our citrus juices. Incredibly light in flavor, these juices aid in detoxification and boost the immune system. Lemon is one of our favorite ingredients to use in juice, as it not only adds an alkalizing component but also mellows out a lot of the more intense flavors of other ingredients without robbing the juices of their important nutritional value.

Something Sweet: These are our favorite fruit juice recipes, which are super easy to make in large quantities and popular with children.

The "Milk" Bar: Many people prefer our recipes for almond, cashew, and rice milks to dairy versions.

Smooth Operator: Everybody loves a smoothie. They are refreshing and delicious, an excellent breakfast or snack, and extra-satisfying, since all of the fiber stays put. If you want to be a smooth operator at home, this is where a blender will come in handy.

Savory and Spicy: You will find some unique savory juice flavors that are not available in stores but which our test kitchen has worked tirelessly to perfect, making savory options available for people who are a bit tired of the sweetness that store-bought juices tend to have. These juices can also be blended with a base such as lightly steamed carrots or broccoli to make light, easily digestible soups that are filled with nutrients.

Elixirs and Flavored Waters: These shots and tonics are designed to promote overall health.

how to use these recipes

At Pressed Juicery, our goal is to be as transparent and simple as possible. We love to laugh, and some of our recipes have clever names, but generally speaking, we are ingredient focused and want what's in the juice to speak for itself. From the beginning, our menu has used three categories: greens, roots, and citrus, with the different varieties designated by a simple numerical system (you know, 1, 2, 3, . . .). This has always made ordering as simple as 1, 2, 3! Our customers tell us they enjoy coming in to our stores and asking for their favorite: Greens 3, Roots 4, and Citrus 2, for example. It makes things easy and clean, just the way we like it. We've kept this tradition alive as much as possible within the pages of this book.

Note that each recipe yields varying quantities of juice, but they are all meant to serve at least one or two people. We encourage you to experiment to see which recipes you want to double or even triple.

As a general rule, if you are using a centrifugal juicer, we recommend drinking juices as soon as possible, but if you must store them in the refrigerator, use an airtight container and store the juice for no longer than 24 hours. If you use a masticating juicer, do not store longer than 48 hours. Smoothies and juices made at home on a hydraulic press or twin-gear juicer can last up to 72 hours. An interesting thing to note is that citrus is a natural preservative; you will notice that when you add citrus fruits such as lemon to your drinks, the flavors will stay better for longer and so will the quality of the juice.

You'll see that our recipes list out the ingredients but don't share specific instructions for juicing and mixing. That's because the juicing process is basically the same for every recipe. We didn't want to repeat it sixty times, so we've outlined below how to juice. Apply these two steps to any and all of the recipes, and you're good to go.

STEP 1: WASH AND PREP YOUR PRODUCE

Most juicers can handle the skin on fruits and veggies, so start by scrubbing them well with water and a fruit and veggie wash, if you'd like (see box below). Citrus fruits like lemons and oranges should be coarsely peeled, meaning that most of the rind should be removed for a more pleasing flavor, but you can leave the pith and some minor bits of rind. Although there are no rules and the rind won't hurt you, most people prefer the flavor of juice when the rind is removed. Cucumbers and ginger should also be peeled, as they have bitter-tasting skin, as should melons, whose rinds are simply too thick to put through a conventional juicer. Root veggies should be soaked or scrubbed with extra elbow grease to get the dirt off.

STEP 2: JUICE

Add your prepped ingredients to your juicer according to the amounts called for in the recipe. There are no rules as to what order to juice them—just pop in your fruits and veggies in one run as you like. The flavors all blend in liquid form regardless. For many recipes, this is your last step. The juices can be enjoyed at room temperature, or if you like them chilled, add a couple of ice cubes.

If you're improvising, add only small amounts of ginger, garlic, and herbs, because a tiny bit packs a strong punch. If you're using a centrifugal juicer, it's a good idea to juice your ingredients once and then put the pulp through the juicer a second time to maximize the amount of juice yielded.

It's as simple as that! Prep the produce and let the machine do the work so you can get your juice on!

CLEANING YOUR FRUITS AND VEGGIES:
The Spray Method versus the Soak Method

SPRAY: Combine 1 cup of water, 2 tablespoons of lemon juice, and 1 cup of vinegar in a clean spray bottle. Gently shake to mix. Spray your produce and let it sit for 1 to 2 minutes, then rinse well with clean water. Store your spray mix in the refrigerator between uses.

SOAK: Combine ¼ cup of lemon juice and 1 cup of vinegar in a bowl. Soak your produce for at least 1 or 2 minutes, then remove and rinse well with clean water. Note: Soak root veggies for 3 to 4 minutes and soak leafy greens for at least 2 minutes; the soak will make your greens more crisp and fresh tasting, too.

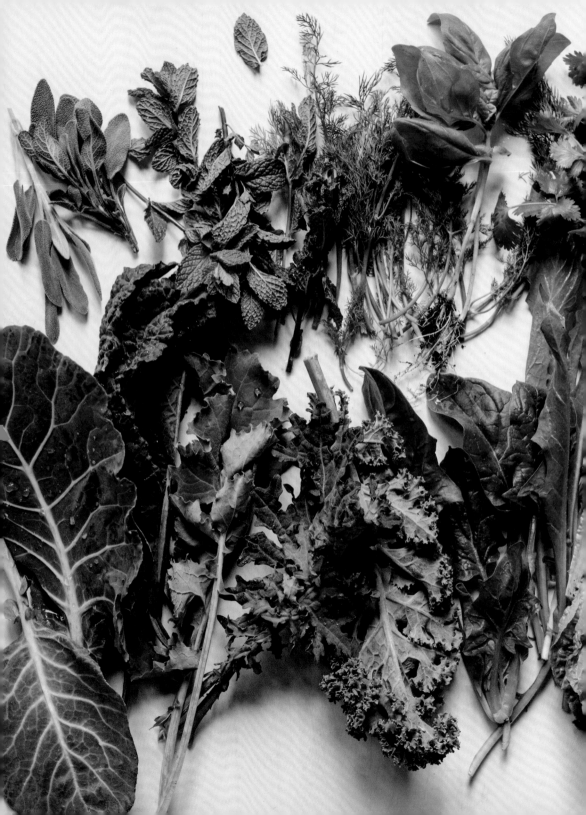

CHAPTER 3

IT'S ALL ABOUT THE GREENS

We like to think of green juice as your gateway drug into the world of healthy living. Greens are nutrition powerhouses, packed with vitamins and minerals that actually aid in energizing and revitalizing the system. And the deep-green jewel tones are a sign that good things are happening, because the natural chemicals that give veggies their luscious hues also provide antioxidants and phytonutrients that support our health, growth, repair, and immune systems.

When our cells are truly fed nutritionally dense foods (not just calorie-dense foods), we experience a kind of energy that we would never get from a protein-packed, processed energy bar. The challenge with leafy greens for some people is that it's hard to eat as much as we should in one meal or even one day. Rumor has it that our ancient ancestors used to walk along picking green vegetables and eating pounds of them each day. Now most of us cannot imagine coming close to eating that much of any type of veggie every day.

The beauty of juicing is that it makes this level of intake possible. You get the vitamins and minerals—and even some of the fiber—from a large amount of produce, but it comes to you in a form that is easy and quick to consume and digest. Green juice is also one of the most alkalizing things you can put into your body—you can immediately feel it working wonders and seemingly calming down your insides as you drink it.

Our team has worked long and hard on the recipes for all of our juices, but we are particularly proud of our greens. They make up the basis for our signature cleanses, but they can also be enjoyed on their own as a great way to start the day, end the day, and everything in between.

As anyone whose life has changed through juicing will tell you, it's all about the greens.

GREENS 1

Leafy green vegetables are especially remarkable because they contain such concentrated amounts of vitamins and minerals. There are barely any carbohydrates in leafy greens, and the carbs that are present digest slowly, which means they won't spike your blood sugar levels. We love having kale in our green juices because of all of its health benefits: it is extremely high in vitamins K, A, C, and E and contains high levels of the minerals manganese, copper, calcium, potassium, iron, and magnesium. Not to mention, it is full of fiber and even contains protein and omega-3 fatty acids. Greens 1 is excellent for preventing disease, promoting cardiovascular health and natural detoxification, and reducing inflammation.

MAKES 1 TO 2 (8-OUNCE) SERVINGS

2 or 3 large kale leaves, to taste

Large handful of spinach

1 head romaine

2 celery stalks

1 large or 2 small cucumbers, peeled

1 small bunch fresh parsley

GREENS 1.5

This is exactly what it sounds like: Greens 1, with a little something extra added. Here we include lemon and lime juices to give our basic green juice a tangy upgrade. One of the star veggies in Greens 1.5 is cucumber. While primarily known for their high water content, cucumbers are rich in vitamins K and C as well as potassium. Cucumbers also contain antioxidants, making them anti-inflammatory and agents for cancer prevention.

MAKES 1 TO 2 (8-OUNCE) SERVINGS

2 or 3 kale leaves, to taste

Large handful of spinach

1 head romaine

2 celery stalks

1 large or 2 small cucumbers, peeled

1 small bunch fresh parsley

½ lemon, peeled

½ lime, peeled

GREENS 2

We fill our green juices with romaine, which is extremely high in vitamins A, K, and C; folate; and the minerals molybdenum, manganese, and potassium. This juice can help you maintain your eye and skin health, not to mention your cardiovascular functioning. In addition, vitamin K is essential for proper blood clotting and bone building. We add a bit of apple juice to this recipe to make it just a little sweet.

MAKES 1 TO 2 (16-OUNCE) SERVINGS

2 or 3 kale leaves, to taste

Large handful of spinach

1 head romaine

2 celery stalks

1 large or 2 small cucumbers, peeled

1 small bunch fresh parsley

1 Fuji apple

½ lemon, peeled

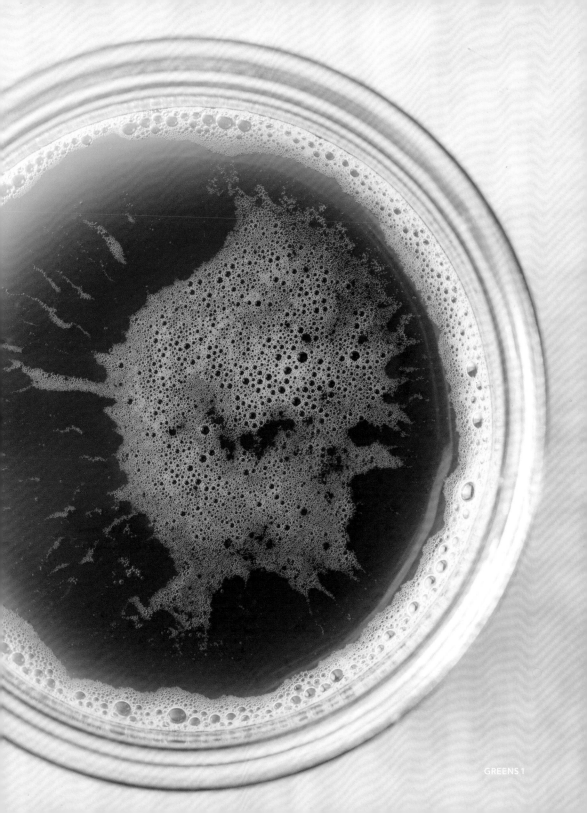

GREENS 3

In this version of green juice, we add ginger to spice things up. The sweetness of the apple, the tart kick of lemon, and the health benefits of the ginger combine really well in what many people tell us is their favorite green juice.

MAKES 1 TO 2 (16-OUNCE) SERVINGS

2 or 3 kale leaves, to taste

Large handful of spinach

1 head romaine

2 celery stalks

1 large or 2 small cucumbers, peeled

1 small bunch fresh parsley

1 Fuji apple

½ lemon, peeled

½-inch piece fresh ginger, peeled

GREENS 4

Watercress is not just for tea sandwiches. Rich in vitamins K, A, and C, as well as the B vitamins, watercress is a valuable antioxidant. In addition, it contains a unique compound called gluconasturtiin, which is believed to promote detoxification of the liver. In this recipe, the spicy green pairs with the coolness of cucumber, the warmth of ginger, and the kick of cayenne for a green juice full of flavor.

MAKES 1 TO 2 (16-OUNCE) SERVINGS

2 cucumbers, peeled

2 celery stalks

1 bunch or large handful of watercress

1 lemon, peeled

½-inch piece fresh ginger, peeled

½ teaspoon cayenne pepper

GREENS 5

A bright, spicy, fresh-tasting way to get your daily greens, this juice is a perfect start your morning. Fennel, which is in the same family as carrots, dill, celery, and parsley, is a good source of vitamin C (as is the orange) and contains essential oils that give it an aniseed smell, which we love! Its fragrance is a nice complement to the juice. Most important, it is useful for digestion and it relaxes the walls of the gut. You could replace the cilantro with ginger to give this juice a different spin.

MAKES 1 TO 2 (16-OUNCE) SERVINGS

Large handful of spinach

1 orange, peeled

½ small fennel bulb

1 head romaine

½ pineapple, skin removed

4 or 5 sprigs fresh cilantro, to taste

GREENS 6

If you enjoy Thai food, you probably already know that lemongrass and cilantro were made for each other. Here, the pair blends beautifully with sweet honeydew, sweet kiwi, and mellow green spinach to round it all out. And lucky for you, cilantro is one of the premier herbs for detoxification and cleansing, especially of heavy metals, which makes it popular among health enthusiasts. In addition, it has traditionally been used for improving cholesterol and blood sugar levels.

MAKES 1 TO 2 (8-OUNCE) SERVINGS

Large handful of spinach

½ honeydew, rind removed

1 kiwi, peeled

2 lemongrass stalks

4 or 5 sprigs fresh cilantro, to taste

GREENS 7

Parsley is best known for its high vitamin K content, making it a key nutrient for blood and bone health. But its volatile oils and flavonoids really make it an interesting herb. The oils are believed to inhibit tumor growth and protect against carcinogens (cancer-causing agents), while its flavonoids protect our cells from damage. Finally, parsley is rich in vitamin C, which can provide arthritis relief.

MAKES 1 TO 2 (8-OUNCE) SERVINGS

Large handful of spinach

1 bunch fresh parsley

4 or 5 sprigs fresh mint, to taste

1 pineapple, skin removed

GREENS 8

Why do we include spinach in so many of our green juices? Because spinach is extremely high in vitamins K, A, and C and the B vitamins, and it contains the minerals manganese, iron, calcium, potassium, phosphorus, and copper. Manganese is essential for bone health and plays a role in connective tissue formation, the proper function of the thyroid and sex hormones, and regulation of blood sugar.

MAKES 1 TO 2 (8-OUNCE) SERVINGS

3 or 4 kale leaves, to taste

Large handful of spinach

2 large carrots

1 grapefruit, coarsely peeled (see box on page 66)

GREENS 9

Rich in vitamins C , K, and A, broccoli also has high levels of B vitamins and the minerals manganese and potassium. Broccoli is part of the cruciferous family, which is renowned for a laundry list of health benefits, most notably its anticancer properties. It also contains a key component that aids in hormone balance, spe- cifically targeting harmful xenoestrogens found in substances such as plastics and conventional meat, dairy, and soy. Finally, it is a powerful anti-inflammatory and detoxifying agent, and it promotes colon and cardiovascular health. This recipe also includes alfalfa sprouts. We love sprouts for their concentrated vitamin content and increased enzyme count.

MAKES 1 TO 2 (8-OUNCE) SERVINGS

Small handful of alfalfa sprouts

1 bunch watercress

6 sprigs fresh parsley

3 kale leaves

3 or 4 florets broccoli, to taste

1 Fuji apple

A WORD ON SPROUTS
BY LAUREN FELTS

Lauren Felts is a certified nutritionist, owner of the health and wellness website the Holy Kale, and author of The Miracle Kidney Cleanse. *She is also the in-house nutritionist at Pressed Juicery. As an advocate for others on their quest for health, Lauren specializes in holistic nutrition, cleansing, and toxin-free living. Her expertise is peppered throughout this book, explaining the amazing health benefits in all of our recipes.*

Sprouts are literally the seed of life, the culmination of every nutrient needed for the growth and maturation of a life-form, so it is no wonder that sprouts are at the top of our list to include in a healthy diet. When a seed sprouts, it activates powerful enzyme systems that create extremely high levels of nutrients, including vitamins, minerals, and antioxidants. The interesting thing is that due to this process, sprouts are richer in nutrients than their matured counterparts. Mother Nature sure knows what she's doing!

One of the most accessible sprouts is alfalfa. Alfalfa sprouts, like other sprouts, are rich in nutrients, but they are most well-known for their saponin content. Saponins are compounds that clinical studies have suggested help protect the human body against cancers and also lower cholesterol levels. Research has also indicated that sapo- nins decrease blood lipids, lower blood glucose response, and can be used in the inhibition of dental cavities and platelet aggregation. That's a long list of benefits for such a small sprout!

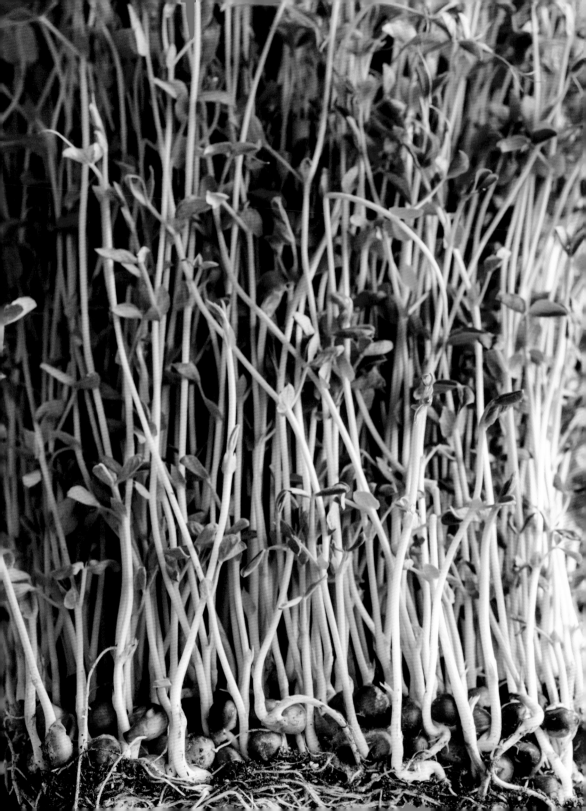

GREENS 10

The smooth, sweet flavors of apple, cucumber, and celery combine with the perfumy, light flavor of fennel in this juice. We add a hint of lime and a kick of ginger, but you can opt for lemon as well. The celery adds some wonderful health benefits. Best known for its high water content, celery is an excellent natural diuretic. And it delivers loads of vitamins, specifically vitamins K and A, as well as folate, potassium, and molybdenum.

MAKES 1 TO 2 (16-OUNCE) SERVINGS

2 small green apples

1 cucumber, peeled

2 or 3 celery stalks, leaves on, to taste

1 fennel bulb and stem

½ lime, peeled

½-inch piece fresh ginger, peeled

GREENS 11

Dandelions are more than just a weed in your backyard; they are actually nutritional powerhouses. More nutrient dense than most veggies in the produce aisle, dandelion greens are antioxidant and diuretic, and they detoxify and cleanse the liver, kidneys, and digestive system.

MAKES 1 TO 2 (8-OUNCE) SERVINGS

3 or 4 dandelion green leaves, to taste

1 large or 2 small cucumbers, peeled

2 celery stalks

½ lemon, peeled

1 small green or red apple

GREENS 12

Collard greens are rich in vitamins K, A, and C and the B vitamins, as well as the minerals calcium, manganese, iron, and magnesium. They are also known for their ability to lower cholesterol, prevent cancer, and act as an anti-inflammatory agent. Here we pair them with green bell peppers for a slightly savory flavor.

MAKES 1 TO 2 (8-OUNCE) SERVINGS

2 cucumbers, peeled

2 green bell peppers

5 or 6 collard green leaves, to taste

3 carrots

2 lemons, peeled

MAKE JUICE, NOT WAR
GREEN JUICE

BY KRIS CARR

Hayden says, "When I was a freshman at NYU, I lived in the college dorms. On my own for the first time, I was suddenly surrounded by bars that never seemed to close, diners that sold greasy fries and burgers twenty-four hours a day, and people who thrived on staying out late and living on potato chips. My health was the last thing on my mind—at first. Soon I realized that my lifestyle was leaving me with very little energy for classes and everything else that mattered to me. Then I met Kris Carr, and she introduced me to a better way to live. This woman saved her own life through healthy eating and living, and she completely changed mine. Kris is a New York Times *best-selling author and cancer activist who educates people about how to eat and drink for maximum health. You may already be familiar with Kris and her Crazy Sexy way of living; if not, give this green juice a try and then get your hands on one of her books!*

Rejuvenating, alkaline green juices are the lifeblood of my Crazy Sexy diet and lifestyle. Juicing your organic fruits and veggies is the best and quickest ways to reduce inflammation (the root cause of most chronic disease) while hydrating your body, drenching your cells in life-giving nutrients, and even repairing your DNA. Yes, you read that correctly. Say hello to boundless energy, glowing skin, clear eyes, improved digestion, and exceptional health and happiness. Say good-bye to toxins, excess weight, sugar cravings, addictions, premature aging, and a lackluster appearance.

How do I know this? My whiskey-tango-foxtrot moment (that's military lingo for WTF?!), getting a diagnosis of incurable stage IV cancer, sparked a deep desire in me to stop holding back and start living like I mean it. Since I couldn't do chemo, radiation, or have surgery (none available), I decided to look outside the box to feel better and participate in my health and happiness. That's when I found juice.

Do this: Drink your fruits and vegetables. Do it daily. Start with one liquid elixir per day and inch up to two or three over time. And as you up your juice intake, feel free to reduce your crap intake. Trust me. This is it. The medicine. The muse. The game changer. It won't let you down. It's my motto and my morning beverage.

MAKES 2 (16-OUNCE) SERVINGS

2 large cucumbers, peeled
Large handful of kale
Large handful of romaine
4 or 5 celery stalks, to taste
1 or 2 big broccoli stems, to taste (for sweetness)
1-inch piece fresh ginger, peeled

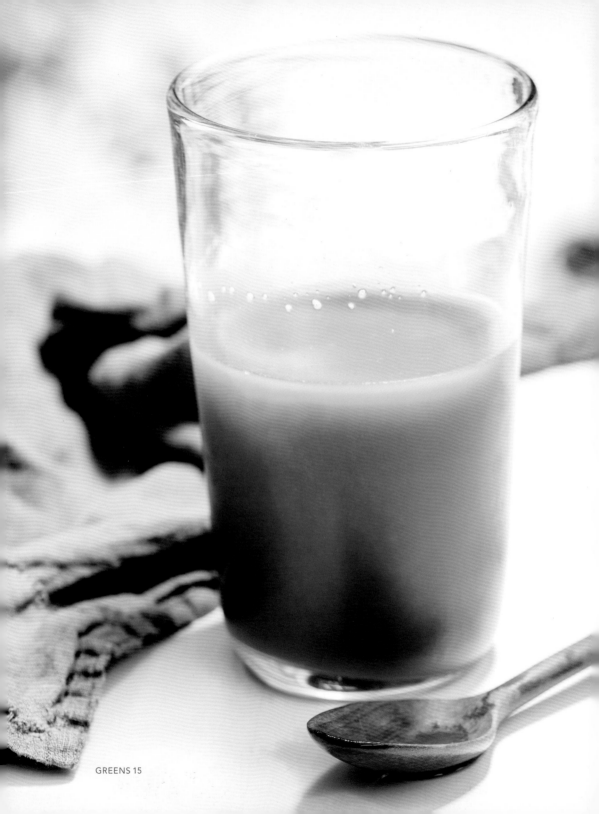

GREENS 13

Cucumber and celery bring the crisp, pear and honeydew bring the sweet, and lemon and ginger bring the bite for a balanced juice that's also a diuretic, an alkalizer, and a taste bud pleaser.

MAKES 1 TO 2 (16-OUNCE) SERVINGS

1 cucumber, peeled
2 celery stalks
1 pear
½ honeydew, rind removed
4 kale leaves
½ lemon, peeled
½-inch piece fresh ginger, peeled

GREENS 14

Spicy and sweet, this sophisticated juice goes double on the herbs and has a touch of apple.

MAKES 1 TO 2 (8-OUNCE) SERVINGS

1 cucumber, peeled
2 celery stalks
1 bunch fresh cilantro
3 or 4 fresh basil leaves, to taste
2 Fuji apples

GREENS 15

Triple leafy greens plus triple fruit equals triple threat. Here we add fennel, celery, and cucumber for a super hydrating juice that is not overly sweet.

MAKES 1 TO 2 (8-OUNCE) SERVINGS

3 celery stalks
1 cucumber, peeled
2 kale leaves
2 Swiss chard leaves
½ small fennel bulb
1 Fuji apple
1 pear
1 lemon, peeled
1 bunch fresh parsley

NATALIA'S GREEN LEMONADE

Carly says, "The first green juice I ever tried contained a bunch of veggies that usually taste harsh on their own—kale, spinach, celery—but when I juiced them together, they were somehow balanced, sweet, refreshing, and honestly delicious! I followed a recipe from *The Raw Food Detox Diet* by Natalia Rose, and it became a staple for me. After experiencing the energizing effects of her juice, I started to slowly replace my daily caffeine fix with it and eventually made healthier choices about what I put on my plate throughout the day. I experienced my taste buds, and shortly after, my life changed as I made a shift toward foods that were truly feeding me. Natalia graciously agreed to let us share my favorite recipe with you. I hope it will inspire you to get on the green bandwagon, too."

MAKES 1 TO 2 (8-OUNCE) SERVINGS

1 head romaine
5 or 6 kale leaves
1 or 2 Fuji apples, to taste

1 lemon, peeled
1 to 2 tablespoons fresh ginger, peeled, to taste (optional)

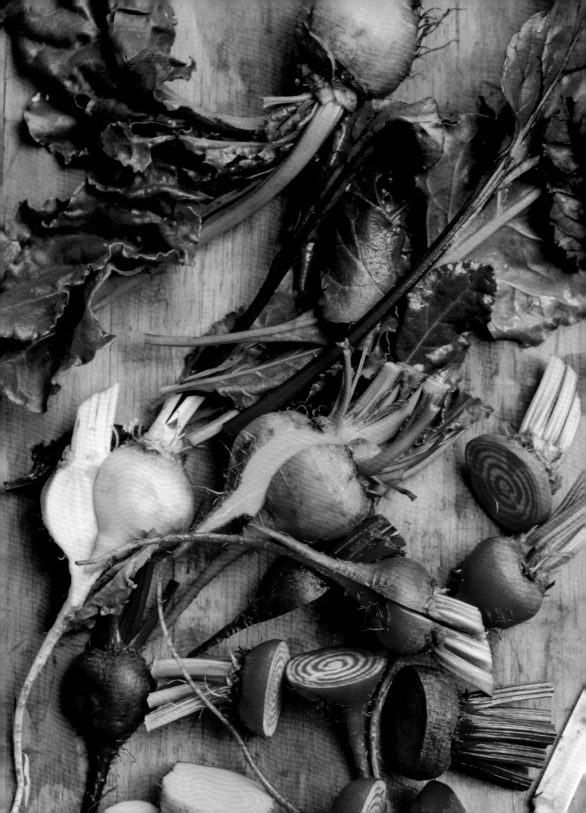

CHAPTER 4

GET BACK TO YOUR ROOTS

Grown deep in the ground, root vegetables like carrots and beets and ginger—that's right, ginger is a root!—absorb high amounts of vitamins and minerals from the soil as well as from the sun through leaves that grow toward the sky. They have distinct, earthy flavors and are packed with fiber and complex carbohydrates, which help sugars be released into the bloodstream more slowly.

The root veggies you have gotten to know and love in Thanksgiving side dishes take on a refreshing new identity when they are turned into juice. The flavors are sweet and milder than you might expect, but still rich and hearty. Greens give us the energy we need to lift us during the day; roots have a very grounding energy that many people find they need, especially during the winter months.

Thinking of food in terms of energy that goes beyond calories is called the energetics of food. The awareness of how our bodies react with foods depending on where the food grew, and how, is something that practices like traditional Chinese medicine and other holistic approaches to health cultivate and teach. Within those practices, food is something deeper than caloric energy. It is used for medicinal purposes and for healing specific ailments.

Think about how you feel at different times of the day, month, or year. Many of us find that we crave specific foods at different times of year (like salads in the summertime or hearty soups and stews in winter). But we are often so distracted with daily life that we may never get to the root of those desires, which may be expressing a deep nutritional and emotional need that our bodies have. Whether or not you've ever thought about food as something that corresponds to your mood, you've surely had cravings for various foods at times. Part of eating well is learning to really listen to your body as it speaks to you and tells you what it needs. We find that when the weather gets cooler, we tend to crave many of our heartier roots recipes; however, any of these can be enjoyed throughout the year.

ROOTS 1

There's just something about beets that makes us feel so darn healthy. Beets contain unique phytonutrients called betalains, which provide support for the body's antioxidants and detoxification process. Beets are known to aid the process of flushing the bad stuff from our liver and kidneys, where many of the body's toxins are stored.

MAKES 1 TO 2 (16-OUNCE) SERVINGS

1 beet (see box below)

3 carrots

3 kale leaves

1 cucumber, peeled

2 celery stalks

1 head romaine

1 bunch fresh parsley

Large handful of spinach

ROOTS 2

Bright and refreshing, carrots and cucumbers have a lovely balance of light and sweet. Carrots are packed with beta-carotene, which gets converted into vitamin A, an essential vitamin for eye health, especially night vision.

MAKES 1 TO 2 (8-OUNCE) SERVINGS

4 or 5 carrots, to taste

1 large cucumber, peeled

Large handful of spinach

1 bunch fresh parsley

ROOTS 3

As you may have noticed, we love ginger around here. The beauty of ginger is that it can be added to almost anything. It's a great complement for both savory and sweet juices, and it adds an amazing dose of health benefits (see page 32). Ginger also tastes lovely on its own with warm water. In this juice, ginger is paired with beets, apple, and lemon for a hot-pink ginger lemonade that is ridiculously delicious. Who needs food coloring when you have gorgeous red beets?

MAKES 1 TO 2 (8-OUNCE) SERVINGS

3 beets (see box below)

1 Fuji apple

½ lemon, peeled

½-inch piece fresh ginger, peeled

HOW TO PREP AND USE BEETS IN JUICE

Scrub your beets well (you don't have to peel them), then cut off their tops (the leafy beet greens make an amazing side dish or an addition to your juice). Because beets do have a good amount of sugar and they are naturally very sweet, a little goes a long way in juice. When you're creating your own juice recipes, start with a small amount of beet and then add more to taste.

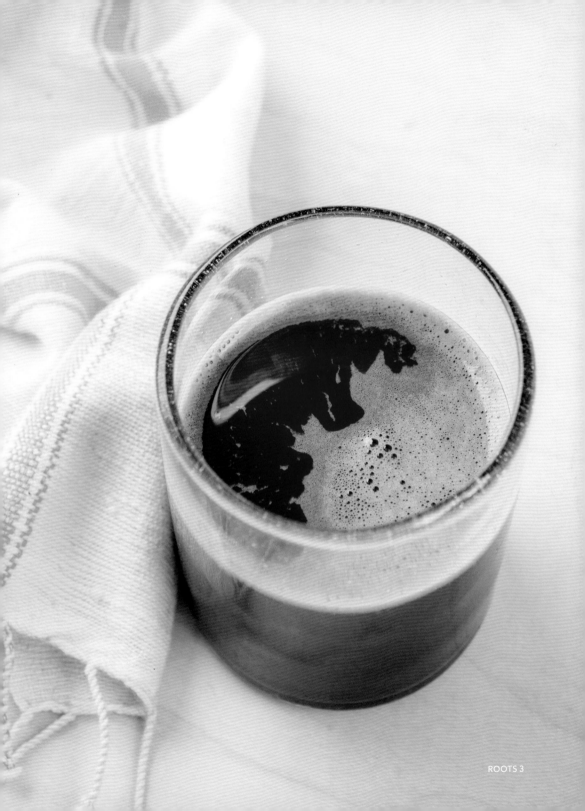

ROOTS 4

Carrot-apple juice is a classic
recipe often found in natural
food stores and health food
restaurants. Here we take it
to a new level by adding, you
guessed it, a hint of ginger.
The flavors balance to create
an earthy, tangy juice that is
perfect any time of day.

**MAKES 1 TO 2 (8-OUNCE)
SERVINGS**

4 carrots
1 Fuji apple
½-inch piece fresh
ginger, peeled

ROOTS 5

If you've never tried burdock root, this is a great introductory recipe. Burdock root is widely used for medicinal purposes in Asia and is a staple of Japanese cuisine. Known as a bitter root, it is a blood purifier, promoting kidney function. Antibacterial and anti-inflammatory, it contains probiotics, which stimulate the growth of healthy bacteria in the gut. Many people drink it in tea and add it to soups, but it is also excellent for juicing. It can be found in many grocery stores.

MAKES 1 TO 2 (8-OUNCE) SERVINGS

Handful of any leafy greens, such as kale, chard, or spinach

½-inch piece fresh ginger, peeled

1 burdock root, about ¼ pound

3 small red or green apples

½ lemon, peeled

ROOTS 6

Apple juice is for kids; apple-celery-burdock root is for grown-ups who like their juice a little more interesting.

MAKES 1 TO 2 (8-OUNCE) SERVINGS

2 Fuji apples

4 celery stalks

1 burdock root, about ¼ pound

ROOTS 7

Like carrots and beets, parsnips take on a totally new personality when you run them through a juicer. While it's not very common to find parsnips in juices, we love their mildly sweet and earthy flavor and find that it adds something unique and unexpected to a juice that you just can't get from your average carrot.

MAKES 1 TO 2 (8-OUNCE) SERVINGS

4 or 5 carrots, to taste

1 cucumber, peeled

2 parsnips

1 lemon, peeled

ROOTS 8

Radishes are not often used in the juicing world. However, their spicy profile kicks up the flavor of any juice with added benefits: they are helpful in mediating stress due to their ability to support the adrenal glands. In addition, the high vitamin C content of radishes helps in the formation of collagen; anyone who's fighting wrinkles will appreciate this. In this recipe, the combination of spicy radishes, bright lime, sweet pear, and cool cucumber makes a fresh and balanced afternoon pick-me-up.

MAKES 1 TO 2 (8-OUNCE) SERVINGS

4 radishes

1 lime, coarsely peeled

1 cucumber, peeled

1 pear

CARROT BREAD

As you will notice once you start getting your juice on, juicing means pulp. A lot of pulp can build up when you extract the juice from your produce. The amount depends on the type of juicer you have, how much produce you are using, and how many times you run it through the machine. When you're finished juicing, don't just toss all that yummy pulp! It is full of nutrition and fiber, and it can be incorporated into some delicious recipes, like this wonderful carrot bread.

MAKES 6 TO 8 SERVINGS (ABOUT 9 PIECES)

1½ cups carrot pulp

4 organic eggs

¼ cup melted organic butter or ghee (clarified butter)

1 cup coconut flour

1 teaspoon baking soda

1 teaspoon cinnamon

½ teaspoon freshly grated nutmeg

Juice of ½ small lemon

1 tablespoon apple cider vinegar

1 teaspoon vanilla extract

1 tablespoon maple syrup

½ cup walnuts (optional)

2 tablespoons raisins (optional)

Preheat the oven to 325°F and place a tray of water in the bottom of the oven. Line an 8 by 8-inch baking dish with parchment paper, leaving a generous trim.

In a mixing bowl, stir together the carrot pulp, eggs, butter, flour, baking soda, cinnamon, and nutmeg and set aside.

In a small bowl, stir together the lemon juice, vinegar, vanilla, and maple syrup. Add this to the carrot mixture and stir until well combined. Stir in the walnuts and raisins.

Pour the batter into the prepared baking dish and smooth the top with a spatula. Bake until the top is golden brown and a toothpick inserted into the middle comes out clean, 50 to 70 minutes.

Allow the bread to cool in the baking dish for about 10 minutes. Remove the bread from the dish and let it cool on a wire rack. Slice and serve warm or at room temperature. The bread will keep in an airtight container at room temperature for up to 3 days.

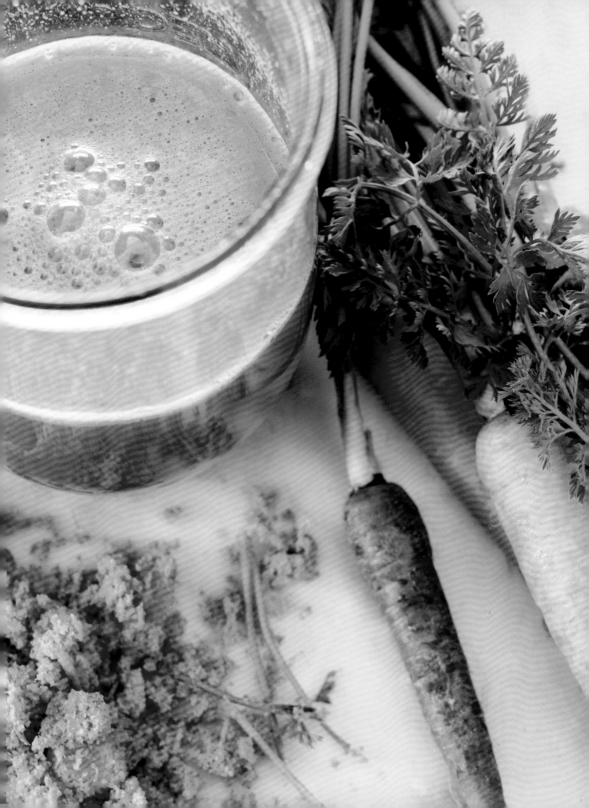

ROOTS 9

Adding beneficial carrots to a heap of greens makes this juice a powerful tonic. Carrots are loaded with antioxidants, which actually makes them a great cancer-preventative agent as well as a tool for improving cardio-vascular health. And greens, as we know, are brilliant detoxifiers and alkalizers.

MAKES 1 TO 2 (8-OUNCE) SERVINGS

2 or 3 carrots, to taste

2 celery stalks

1 cucumber, peeled

3 or 4 dandelion green leaves with stems, to taste

1 bunch fresh parsley

ROOTS 10

This sweet roots drink takes on an earthy tone with the introduction of nutrient-rich parsnip. Parsnips are deli-cious, but we also love these powerful root veggies for their high nutritional content; they are packed with vita-mins K, C, and folate, better known as folic acid, which is part of the vitamin B family.

MAKES 1 TO 2 (8-OUNCE) SERVINGS

1 parsnip

2 carrots

1 beet (see box on page 54)

1 red or green apple

ROOTS 11

As soon as we added pars-nips to our juices (see Roots 7 and Roots 10), we realized that we needed to add some turnips to the mix. Turnips are extremely rich in vitamin C, and their green leaves are a rich source of lutein, an antioxidant, and vitamin A. Here, fennel and apple add some sweetness.

MAKES 1 TO 2 (8-OUNCE) SERVINGS

1 turnip bulb and greens

3 parsnips

1 green apple

¼ or ½ fennel bulb, to taste

ROOTS 12

This juice has got it all. Hearty carrots and mild celery are balanced with apple, lemon, and ginger. Plus we added a garlic clove for a surprising twist. If you like this juice, you'll love what's coming up ahead in our savory section (see chapter 9).

MAKES 1 TO 2 (8-OUNCE) SERVINGS

2 stalks celery

2 carrots

1 clove garlic

1 Fuji apple

½ lemon, peeled

½-inch piece fresh ginger

ROOTS 13

A sweet combination of three of our favorite ingredients, this juice is a crowd-pleaser. While the flavor of the oranges stands out, the beets and carrots add some extra nutrition and beautiful color. We give it to our kids for breakfast in place of classic OJ, and they don't complain!

MAKES 1 TO 2 (8-OUNCE) SERVINGS

2 beets (see box on page 54)

4 carrots

2 oranges, peeled

ROOTS 14

When we're talking about juicing, we don't usually include potatoes. Although regular potatoes are night-shade vegetables (see page 115) and we don't recom-mend eating them during a cleanse, sweet potatoes are *not* part of this group and actually contain many excellent health benefits. We love sweet potatoes for their beta-carotene and vitamin C content. Although they are starchy when you eat them, here you are left with just the light, sweet juice of the potato. Scrub them well and cut them into quarters before running them through your juicer.

MAKES 1 TO 2 (8-OUNCE) SERVINGS

1 sweet potato

2 carrots

½ pineapple, skin removed

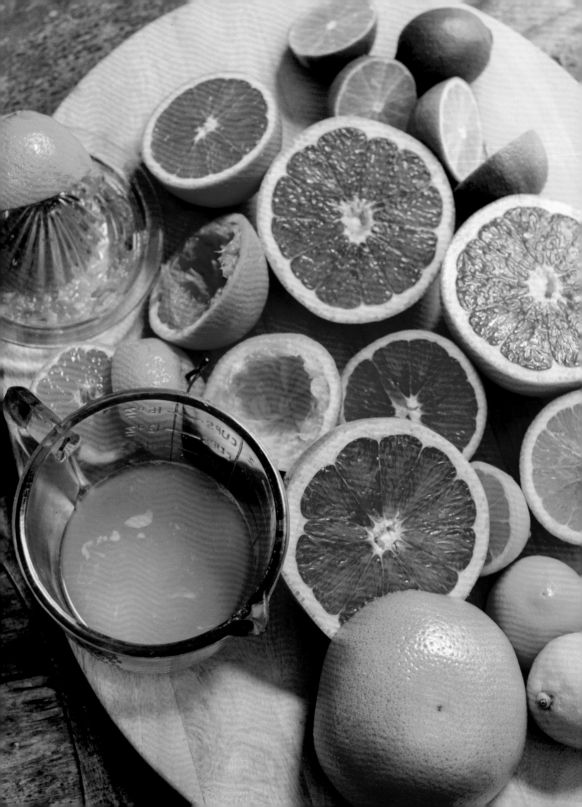

CHAPTER 5

CITRUS APPEAL

At Pressed Juicery, our line of citrus juices are almost as popular as our greens. The versatility of the flavors gives you different options for when you're sick and need a boost of vitamin C, when you want an added dose of hydration after an intense workout, or as a detoxifying tonic that replenishes after a carb-loaded weekend. Although most people are used to seeing orange juice as the base of fruit drinks, there is much more to great-tasting, healthy juice than that good old breakfast staple.

A powerful fruit, lemons are one of the most healing foods you can consume. From an alkalinity standpoint, they are really high on the scale. Most people assume that because lemons are acidic tasting, they must not be alkalizing. In reality, the citric acid in lemons is actually a "weak" acid, and when balanced with the fruit's alkaline minerals, the citric acid is easily eliminated and an alkaline ash is left in the body. Thus, while the food itself may be "acidic," what matters is the effect it has on the body once it is metabolized.

As we've discussed (see page 14), because harmful, disease-causing agents cannot live in an alkaline environment, it is very important to include an array of alkalizing foods in your diet. Lemons are also antiseptic, and a great immune booster. The citric acid content of lemons is a detoxifying agent for the gall-bladder and kidneys. We've said it before, and we'll say it again: water with lemon juice, honey, and apple cider vinegar is our favorite way to start the day. Drink it at room temperature or even heated if you need to soothe a sore throat. Not only does lemon taste refreshing, but it also gives your obligatory water intake extra nutritional value.

There are so many types of citrus fruits, and we love them all because they're loaded with vitamin C and contain pectin fiber, which is an appetite suppressant. Interestingly, apples also contain pectin, and when they are combined with citrus, the resulting juices help stave off hunger pangs, especially for people who are cleansing.

Read on for some of our most crowd-pleasing recipes, packed with oranges, grapefruit, tangerines, limes, and lemons galore.

CITRUS 1

Arguably one of the simplest drinks to make, this spicy lemonade has definitely made its way into the spotlight in the last few years as public interest in cleansing has increased. Even some sections of the grocery store now have displays dedicated to the ingredients needed to put together the Master Cleanse. The Master Cleanse, aka the Lemonade Diet, gained popularity a few decades ago as a weight-loss and detoxification plan. While we don't promote a diet strictly made up of these ingredients, we do find that purified water with lemon juice and cayenne is a great addition to a regimen that also includes nutritionally dense vegetable juices. Cayenne contains capsaicin, which has been found to stimulate the circulatory system and regulate blood sugar. Cayenne is also known to boost the metabolism in the immediate hours after it is consumed, helping the body burn fat.

This drink is a staple in our cleanse program, as well as our daily diets. It hydrates, refreshes, and detoxifies—and trust us, it tastes great, too! Juice the lemon, then stir the juice into the water and add the cayenne.

MAKES 1 (8-OUNCE) SERVING

1 lemon, peeled

8 ounces purified water

½ teaspoon cayenne pepper (or ½ dropperful of liquid cayenne pepper extract)

Note: We recommend that you drink this without added sweetener, but if you are craving something to balance out the tart taste of the lemon, add a bit of stevia or low-glycemic coconut sugar to taste.

CITRUS 2

One unique characteristic of pineapple that makes it one of our favorite ingredients is an enzyme called bromelain. We are huge fans of enzymes because they are an integral part of almost every function in the body, from digestion to energy creation. Bromelain is used therapeutically to improve protein digestion, reduce inflammation, reduce excessive blood coagulation, and prevent tumor growth.

MAKES 1 TO 2 (8-OUNCE) SERVINGS

⅓ pineapple, skin removed

1 green apple

4 or 5 sprigs fresh mint, to taste

1 lemon, peeled

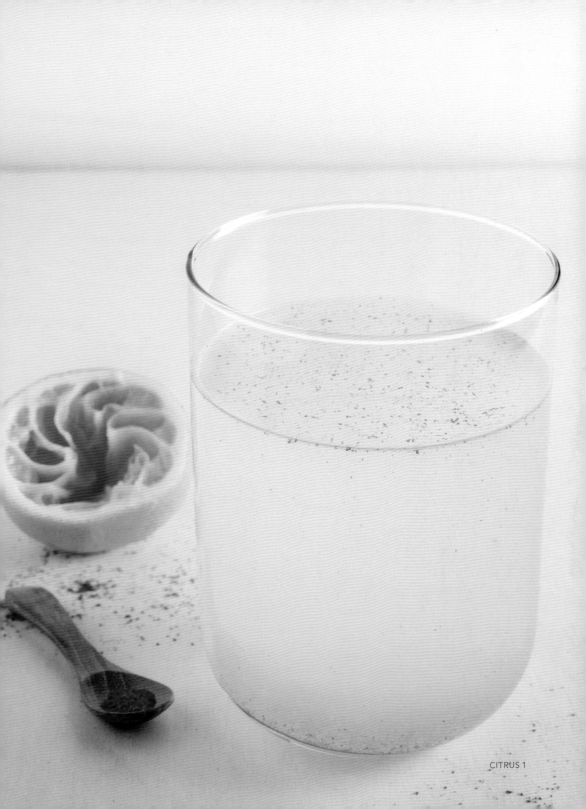

CITRUS 1

CITRUS 3

Why start the day with a plain old orange juice? One of our simplest and most delicious combinations, this grapefruit-mint juice packs a nutritional punch thanks to the incredible power of grapefruit. Aside from being an excellent source of vitamin C, pink and ruby red grapefruits are packed with lycopene, a very powerful antioxidant (also found in tomatoes and green tea) that has been found to help prevent LDL (bad cholesterol) from damaging artery walls. It also contains the soluble fiber called pectin that not only lowers total cholesterol but also is beneficial for lowering triglycerides, which is essential for cardiovascular health, and helps the body fight hunger. For that reason, grapefruit is commonly included in weight-loss regimens.

MAKES 1 TO 2 (8-OUNCE) SERVINGS

1 pink or ruby red grapefruit, peeled (see box below)

Small handful of fresh mint leaves

CITRUS 4

This is one of our most popular and refreshing menu items. What's not to like? The cucumber has a high water content for hydration; the aloe juice is high in antioxidants and aids in digestion and the elimination of toxins; and the coconut water contains electrolytes, so some people use it as a natural hangover remedy. We recommend buying fresh, raw coconut water, but if you can't get your hands on it, add grapefruit juice and some extra cucumber. Be creative!

MAKES 1 TO 2 (16-OUNCE) SERVINGS

1 cucumber, peeled

1/3 pineapple, skin removed

1/2 lemon, peeled

1/2 cup coconut water

1/4 cup aloe vera juice

A WARNING ABOUT GRAPEFRUIT

If you take prescription drugs, it is a good idea to consult your doctor before consuming grapefruits, especially when concentrated into juice. Certain drugs become more potent when combined with grapefruit, and the body has a more difficult time breaking down these pharmaceuticals. More likely than not, you won't have anything to worry about, but in our opinion it's better to be safe than sorry.

CITRUS 5

One of our original best sell-
ers, this apple-lemon-ginger
juice is rich in phytonutrients
called polyphenols, which
prevent blood sugar spikes.
The apples have a high fiber
content and are rich in pectin, a soluble fiber that helps
normalize cholesterol, prevent cardiovascular disease,
and stave off hunger pangs.
This is another way to make
apple juice into a grown-up
favorite.

MAKES 1 TO 2 (8-OUNCE)
SERVINGS

1 Fuji apple

1 Granny Smith apple

1 lemon, peeled

½-inch piece fresh ginger,
peeled

CITRUS 6

A little bit of extra spice is
always nice. Here we add
cayenne pepper and ginger
for a punch of health benefits. People who consume
cayenne sometimes say they
can literally *feel* it working,
giving them a boost that
energizes as it replenishes.
Our customers tell us they
like to heat this one up in the
winter and drink it as a tea to
support their immune system
and fight off seasonal colds.

MAKES 1 TO 2 (8-OUNCE)
SERVINGS

1 Fuji apple

1 green apple

1 lemon, peeled

1-inch piece fresh ginger,
peeled

½ teaspoon cayenne pepper

CITRUS 7

Also known as the Green
Alkalizer, this juice is a spin
on Citrus 6 that includes
the addition of hydrating
cucumber.

MAKES 1 TO 2 (8-OUNCE)
SERVINGS

1 cucumber, peeled

1 green apple

1 lemon, peeled

½-inch piece fresh ginger,
peeled

½ teaspoon cayenne pepper

CITRUS 8

Grapefruit, celery, and
ginger combine to get your
metabolism into gear and
(mildly) suppress the appetite. We sip on this between
meals, and sometimes even
add a dash of cinnamon!

MAKES 1 TO 2 (8-OUNCE)
SERVINGS

1 grapefruit, peeled (see box
on page 66)

3 celery stalks

½-inch piece fresh ginger,
peeled

Pinch of cinnamon (optional)

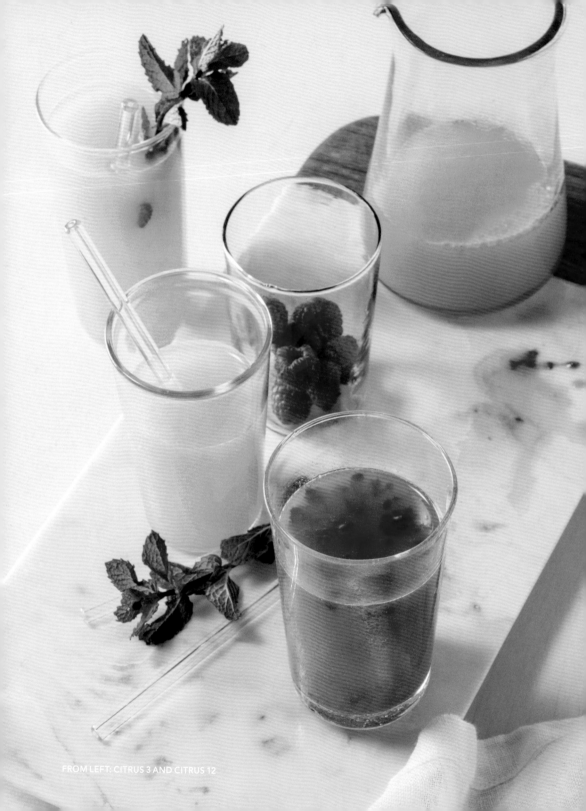

FROM LEFT: CITRUS 3 AND CITRUS 12

CITRUS 9

Who doesn't love orange and pineapple together? We add some celery for its mild veggie flavor and to boost the benefits!

MAKES 1 TO 2 (16-OUNCE) SERVINGS

1 lemon, peeled
1 orange, peeled
½ pineapple, skin removed
3 celery stalks

CITRUS 10

The perfect combination of sweet and tart, this juice always shows up on our menu in late spring or early summer during cherry season. Sweet cherries contain vitamin A and melatonin, a hormone that is naturally secreted in the pineal gland in our brain. It is known for regulating sleep, fighting jet lag, and even slowing down the aging process!

MAKES 1 TO 2 (8-OUNCE) SERVINGS

2 oranges, peeled
1 lime, peeled
15 sweet cherries

CITRUS 11

It is a well-known fact that blueberries are antioxidant powerhouses, and we've yet to meet anyone who doesn't love their flavor as well. In fact, blueberries are considered a superfood because they have a low sugar content and contain a lot of fiber as well as a large amount of cancer-fighting antioxidants. There's nothing we don't love about blueberries, and here we use them to liven up a classic pineapple-orange juice.

MAKES 1 TO 2 (16-OUNCE) SERVINGS

2 oranges, peeled
½ pineapple, skin removed
1 cup blueberries

CITRUS 12

One of our favorite raspberry facts is that they contain high levels of the phytonutrients ellagic acid and anthocyanins. These antioxidant compounds are antiaging and anti-inflammatory. Although they are tiny fruits, raspberries contain significant amounts of these phytonutrients, which can protect the body from disease and chronic illness.

MAKES 1 TO 2 (8-OUNCE) SERVINGS

2 oranges, peeled
1 tangerine, peeled
1 cup raspberries

CITRUS 13

A member of the gourd family, cantaloupe is packed with nutrition. It delivers extremely high amounts of vitamins A and C and beta-carotene. Pairing it with spinach, which contains high levels of zinc, allows the body to utilize the maximum amount of vitamin A present in the cantaloupe. This juice combination has the added upside of making our skin look super radiant; that's pretty amazing!

MAKES 1 TO 2 (16-OUNCE) SERVINGS

2 oranges, peeled
½ canteloupe, rind removed
Handful of spinach
1 cucumber, peeled

CITRUS 14

We added one of our favorite herbs, fresh mint, to complement the flavor of this juice. Mint is known for its ability to quell an uneasy stomach or to freshen breath, but it also contains antimicrobial properties. Therefore, mint can be helpful in preventing the growth of harmful bacteria in the body. We also love it for its cooling and stomach-soothing properties. As an added bonus, it is a natural stimulant that makes us feel energized and lifts our mood.

MAKES 1 TO 2 (8-OUNCE) SERVINGS

2 oranges, peeled
1 tangerine, peeled
½ lemon, peeled
Large handful of fresh mint leaves
2 celery stalks

Variation: Leave out the celery, and you'll have a simple, tangy juice with a hint of mint.

CITRUS 15

This juice blend will make your taste buds very happy. We love the balance of earthy roots; bright, tangy citrus; and the green goodness of spinach and celery to finish it off. Drink this juice a couple of times a week, and your body will thank you.

MAKES 1 TO 2 (16-OUNCE) SERVINGS

2 grapefruits, peeled (see box on page 66)
2 carrots
1 beet (see box on page 54)
2 celery stalks
Handful of spinach
½-inch piece of fresh ginger, peeled

CITRUS 16

The combination of grapefruit and orange cuts the intense flavor of the parsley and watercress, creating a subtle blend with a not-so-subtle boost of vitamins.

MAKES 1 TO 2 (16-OUNCE) SERVINGS

2 grapefruits, peeled (see box on page 66)
2 oranges, peeled
Handful of watercress
1 bunch fresh parsley

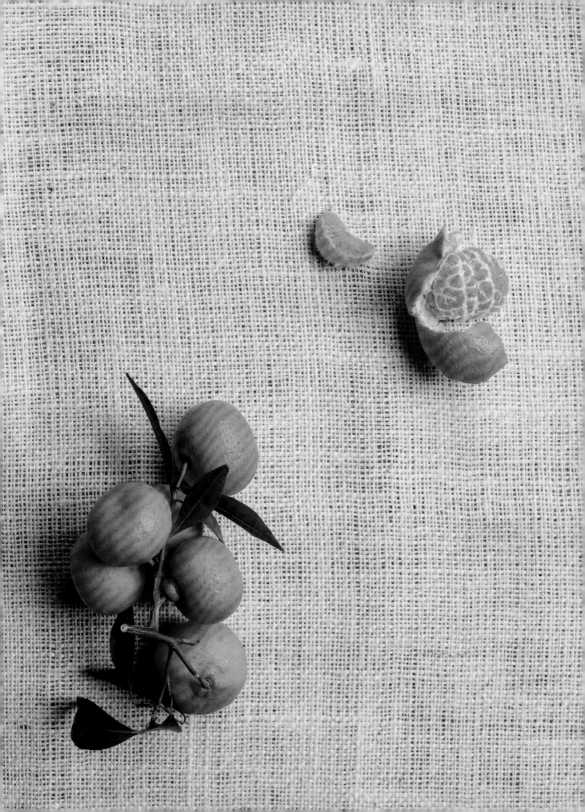

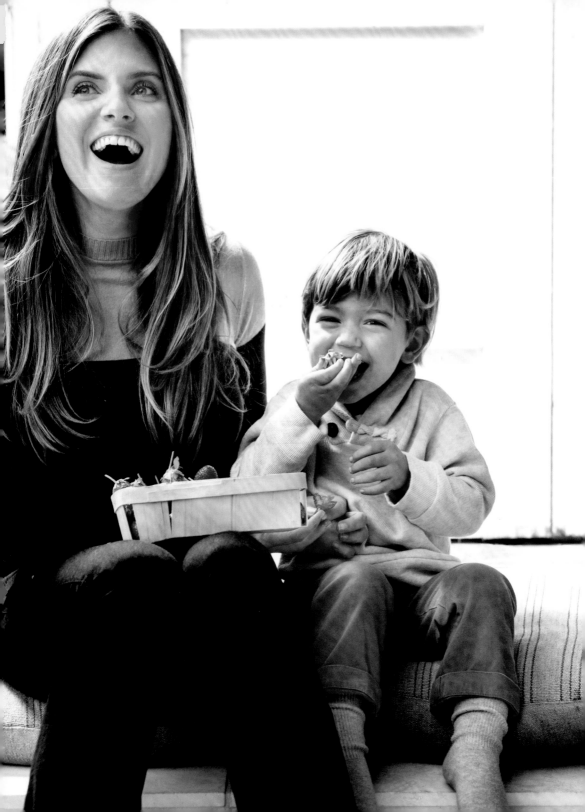

CHAPTER 6

SOMETHING SWEET

Most of the fruit juices on our menu live within our citrus category; however, we do have a few additional favorite combinations that we wanted to share with you. We don't recommend drinking these as part of a cleanse since you are usually cutting out the sugar and focusing on veggie-based juices while cleansing (see more about cleansing on page 109). But these recipes are great for kids, parties, and everyday life. We've also given you some fantastic nutritional reasons to drink these up!

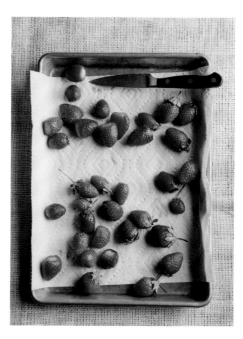

WATERMELON MINT

Watermelon's reputation as the perfect hydrating summer fruit is not without substantiation. Watermelon is 92 percent water, making it one of the top choices for naturally cleansing the body, especially the kidneys. Watermelon is also rich in lycopene (the antioxidant found in tomatoes), which is beneficial for bone and cardiovascular health. Watermelon is also super easy to juice. This one makes a pretty big serving, so put it in a pitcher and don't be afraid to share it.

MAKES 8 TO 10 (8-OUNCE) SERVINGS

1 watermelon, rind removed (see box on page 76)
Handful of fresh mint

WATERMELON, PINEAPPLE, STRAWBERRY, BLUEBERRY, LEMON

This juice simply tastes like vacation, but lucky for us, it's got plenty of benefits to boot! Ranked as two of the best sources of antioxidants, strawberries and blueberries play an important role in protecting our cells from damage. Additionally, it is speculated that the polyphenols found in strawberries regulate blood sugar responses even when consuming white sugars (which we try not to consume very often!).

MAKES 6 TO 8 (8-OUNCE) SERVINGS

½ watermelon, rind removed (see box on page 76)
½ pineapple, rind removed
8 strawberries
1 cup blueberries
½ lemon, peeled

WATERMELON ORANGE PINEAPPLE

It's no secret that oranges are one of the best ways to get your daily dose of vitamin C. It is imperative for maintaining a strong immune system, improving healing time, and supporting the adrenal glands. In this juice, we pair oranges with watermelon and pineapple for a tropical treat. Don't be afraid to put an umbrella in your glass and drink to your health.

MAKES 6 TO 8 (8-OUNCE) SERVINGS

½ watermelon, rind removed (see box on page 76)
2 oranges, peeled
½ pineapple, skin removed

WATERMELON MINT

APPLE, PEAR, MELON, GRAPES, MINT

Melons come in many shapes, sizes, and flavors and contain a large number of nutrients. One of our favorite reasons to eat and drink melon is its high carotenoid content. Carotenoids convert into vitamin A, which not only improves vision, but also is key for reproductive health, bone development, and beautiful skin. In this juice, we pair melon with grapes, apple, pear, and mint—a fruit salad through a straw! Grapes make this combination a perfect grown-up grape juice. While they can be incredibly sweet, they are actually a low-glycemic fruit, meaning they are low in sugar; they are also rich in resveratrol, one of the most effective anti-inflammatory nutrients, which also shows promise in its ability to promote longevity by expressing our antiaging genes.

MAKES 8 TO 10 (8-OUNCE) SERVINGS

2 Fuji apples

1 pear

1 cantaloupe or honeydew melon, rind removed

Handful of red grapes

Small handful of fresh mint leaves

APPLE, STRAWBERRY, LIME

This juice is a best seller in our shops. We love the tanginess that the lime and strawberries add to the apple juice. During the summertime, we pour this juice into ice-pop molds and keep them in the freezer in our office. Everyone goes nuts for them.

MAKES 1 TO 2 (8-OUNCE) SERVINGS

2 Fuji or Pink Lady apples

10 strawberries

1 lime, peeled

DON'T THROW AWAY THE RIND

Watermelon rind contains a compound that produces antioxidant effects. It also has antifungal properties, and we have heard it referred to in the health and wellness world as nature's answer to Viagra—but don't quote us on that one!

To juice watermelon rind, simply chop it into pieces small enough to fit through your juicer. The bitterness of the rind actually becomes quite mild after it has been juiced. Add half a lime to make it taste more interesting if you like.

APPLE, PAPAYA, PEACH, GINGER

Low in calories and packed with nutrients and flavor, peaches are a good source of vitamins A and C and the antioxidant group flavonoids. This is one of our favorite ways to get our daily dose of potassium, a vital mineral for cardiovascular health, as well as the more elusive fluoride. Fluoride is a mineral that is necessary for keeping our teeth strong and preventing and even reversing tooth decay and therefore cavities.

MAKES 1 TO 2 (8-OUNCE) SERVINGS

2 Fuji or Pink Lady apples

1 papaya

1 peach

½-inch piece of fresh ginger, peeled

GRAPEFRUIT, GUAVA, KIWI

Guava is a tropical super-fruit that produces sweet juice and has a high copper content. Copper is a mineral that helps the body produce the skin pigment melanin. Melanin protects our bodies from ultraviolet rays and our nerves from damage, but its most notable effect is its ability to improve thyroid function. Guava is a great food for improving metabolism and aiding in weight loss. In this juice, we pair guava with kiwi, which contains a very high amount of vitamin C, antioxidants, and fiber. We also add grapefruit for extra juice and nutrition.

MAKES 1 TO 2 (8-OUNCE) SERVINGS

1 ruby red grapefruit, peeled (see box on page 66)

1 guava, peeled

2 kiwis, peeled

MANGO, APPLE, STRAWBERRY

Mango is a delicious tropical fruit that is often eaten green with salt and lime juice. But for juicing, you want mangoes that are fully ripe and ready. Mangoes are high in vitamins A and C, and also in fiber and enzymes that aid in digestion. Because mangoes do not always produce a large amount of juice, we add some apples and strawberries to this mix.

MAKES 1 TO 2 (8-OUNCE) SERVINGS

1 ripe mango, skin removed

2 Fuji or Pink Lady apples

8 strawberries

Variation: For a tropical treat, add ½ pineapple, without its skin, to the mix.

PINEAPPLE, BEET, PEAR, GINGER

Along with being a tasty addition to our green juices, pear is one of our favorite fruits for its flavonoid content, which has a lot of promise for improving insulin sensitivity and decreasing diabetes risk and weight gain. An unusual component of pears is cinnamic acid. Cinnamic acid has shown promise in studies to reduce the risk of esophageal, gastric, and colorectal cancer. This juice is extra sweet, so we add ginger for a dose of spice and to balance things out.

MAKES 1 TO 2 (16-OUNCE) SERVINGS

½ pineapple, skin removed

1 beet (see box on page 54)

2 pears

½-inch piece of fresh ginger, peeled

PINEAPPLE, BEET, PEAR, GINGER

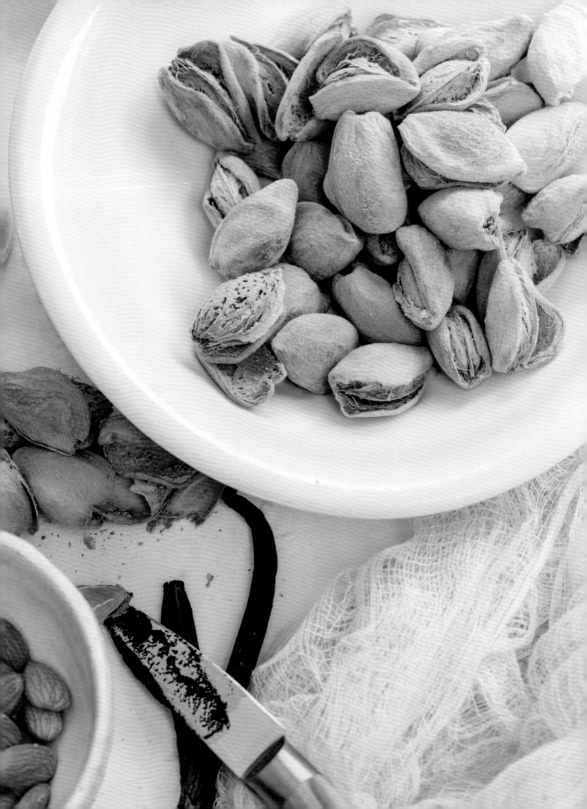

CHAPTER 7

THE "MILK" BAR

So many people these days are discovering that they are allergic to or have sensitivities to dairy products. We noticed such a huge difference in our own health when we began to eliminate it from our diets. In place of dairy, you can purchase milk alternatives like almond and rice milk products, but these are often filled with additives and preservatives. We like to make our own milks; it's easy and they are much healthier.

Almond milk has become a staple of our cleanse program because almonds are packed with protein, fiber, and omega-3 and omega-6 fatty acids. If you have nut allergies, brown rice is a great alternative. In fact, all of the recipes in this chapter can be made with other nuts or brown rice instead of almonds. Just follow the methodology explained in Make Your Own Almond Milk and voilà! Spiced cashew milk, Brazil nut milk, vanilla rice milk . . . whatever your pleasure.

make your own almond milk

Soak your almonds at least overnight, and for as long as two nights. This is a key element to making a great-tasting and healthy beverage; the longer the nuts are soaked, the creamier the results will be. And soaked almonds are much easier to digest.

You will need containers for soaking and storing, a high-speed blender (see page 89) or food processor (although we prefer a high-speed blender because it makes a smoother, less gritty milk), and a nut milk bag (see the Resources, page 144) or at least two layers of cheesecloth.

INGREDIENTS

- Raw, organic almonds
- Purified water for soaking and for blending

FOR SOAKING THE NUTS

- 2 cups of water to every ½ cup of almonds

FOR BLENDING THE NUT MILK

- 2 cups of water to every 1 cup of almonds

- 1 cup of almonds and 2 cups of water = 2 cups of almond milk

- 2 cups of almonds and 4 cups of water = 4 cups of almond milk

Add the desired amount of almonds to a container with the required amount of purified water for soaking (see For Soaking the Nuts, page 81). Cover and soak for 1 to 2 days, then drain the almonds, rinse them with fresh water, and drain again.

Place the soaked almonds in your blender with the required amount of purified water (see For Blending the Nut Milk, page 81). Pulse the blender at low speed, and then increase the speed to the highest setting and blend until smooth, about 2 minutes. You know you're on the right track when the almonds have formed a fine meal and the water is cloudy and white. (If you're using a food processor, this step will take about twice as long.) Once the almonds and water are smooth, add sweeteners or other flavorings according to the recipes (see page 84).

Place a nut milk bag or cheesecloth over the milk container. Wash your hands thoroughly and then strain the almond mixture through the nut milk bag using your hands to squeeze the mixture through the bag. Store the milk in a sealed container in the refrigerator for up to 2 days.

ALMOND MEAL COOKIES

Use the almond meal left from making almond milk in this high-protein, fiber-filled cookie recipe. These can be eaten raw or baked. Use the almond meal from Vanilla Almond Milk (page 84), which is already naturally sweetened.

MAKES 12 TO 16 COOKIES

1 cup almond meal

¼ cup coconut oil

4 to 6 tablespoons almond butter, at room temperature

Grade B maple syrup (optional)

Raw slivered almonds, vegan chocolate chips, chia seeds, or raisins, for topping (optional)

Spread out the almond meal on a baking sheet and let it dry for 2 hours. Pulse the dried meal in a food processor until it has the consistency of flour.

Add the coconut oil, 4 tablespoons of the almond butter, and a bit of maple syrup (to taste) to the food processor and blend until the dough comes together. Add the remaining 2 tablespoons of almond butter if necessary for blending.

Using a tablespoon, scoop balls of batter onto a baking sheet. Add the toppings by pressing them into the top of each dough ball.

If you prefer to eat the cookies raw, pop the baking sheet in the freezer for 15 minutes to let the cookies harden, and then enjoy.

To bake, preheat the oven to 275°F. Bake for 20 minutes, until golden on top. Remove the cookies from the oven and transfer to wire racks to cool. The raw cookies can be stored in an airtight container in the refrigerator, and the baked cookies can be stored in an airtight container at room temperature, for up to 3 days.

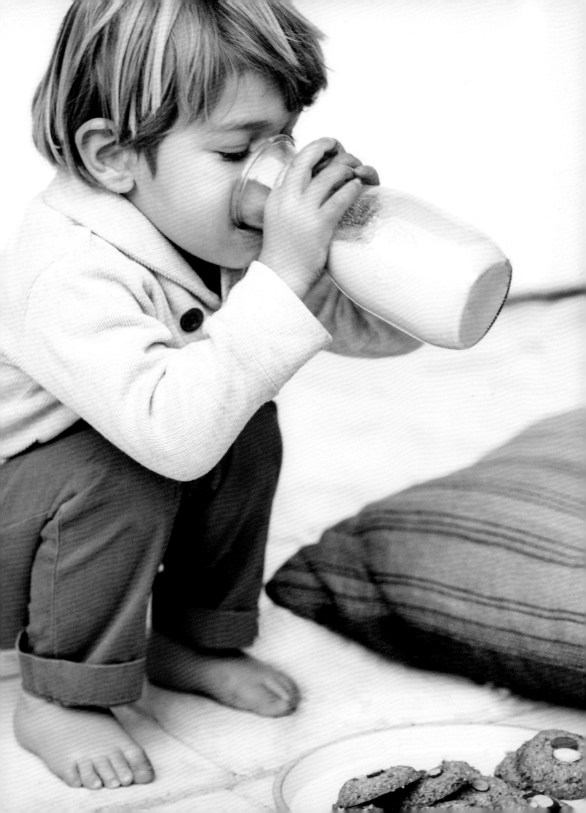

TRADITIONAL ALMOND MILK

This basic almond milk is smooth and mild and so versatile that you can add it to just about anything in place of regular milk—from cereal to a sweet snack.

MAKES ABOUT 2 (8-OUNCE) SERVINGS

1 cup raw, organic almonds

2 cups purified water

VANILLA ALMOND MILK

This is one of our most popular menu items. When cleansing, this is the last drink you have at the end of each day, and our customers tell us they love it. Remember to blend the almonds and water as noted on page 82. Once the consistency is smooth, add the rest of the ingredients and blend again until smooth, then strain.

MAKES ABOUT 2 (8-OUNCE) SERVINGS

1 cup raw, organic almonds

2 cups purified water

½ teaspoon Celtic sea salt

Seeds from ½ fresh vanilla bean (see box below), or ½ teaspoon pure vanilla extract

1 date, pitted (optional)

CHOCOLATE ALMOND MILK

Your kids won't know the difference!

MAKES ABOUT 2 (8-OUNCE) SERVINGS

1 cup raw, organic almonds

2 cups purified water

¼ teaspoon Celtic sea salt

1 tablespoon raw cacao powder

1 date, pitted (optional)

SPICED ALMOND MILK

This is our replacement for holiday eggnog.

MAKES ABOUT 2 (8-OUNCE) SERVINGS

1 cup raw, organic almonds

2 cups purified water

¼ teaspoon Celtic sea salt

½ teaspoon ground cinnamon

½ teaspoon ground cardamom

A NOTE ABOUT VANILLA

While it's often easiest to use vanilla extract, there is something so special about fresh vanilla bean. We use it in all of our almond milk, and we believe you can really taste a difference. To extract the seeds, simply take a fresh vanilla bean pod and split it lengthwise down the middle. Scrape the seeds out of the pod and add them to your recipe.

CHOCOLATE ALMOND MILK

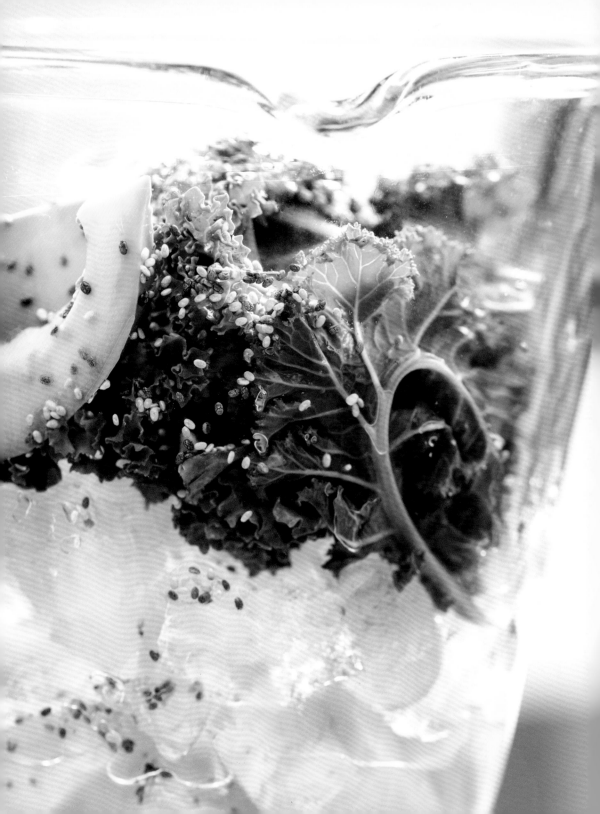

CHAPTER 8

SMOOTH OPERATOR

While we don't make traditional smoothies in most of our stores, we do make them at home, and we know that many people like to add smoothies or shakes to their cleanse programs or simply to their breakfast or lunch routines. When you drink a smoothie instead of a juice, you get added fiber from the fruits and veggies that is sometimes lost in the juicing process. Smoothies are generally more filling, too, and work better than juices as a meal replacement. If you've read through the pantry section (see page 24), you already know how much goodness is packed into the ingredients in these smoothies.

There are so many ways to make smoothies: use all fruits, all vegetables, or a mix of the two; add fresh, frozen, or cooked produce; use a variety of bases for a lighter or creamier smoothie; or make savory smoothies. Although we use ice cubes in most of these recipes, you can replace the ice cubes with a frozen version of any of the fruits and vegetables. For instance, remove the ice and use frozen raspberries in a recipe that calls for fresh raspberries. The idea is to make sure you can taste the ice-cold goodness in your smoothie.

As with the juices, all recipes are designed to make at least one or two servings, but each one yields a slightly different amount. You can simply place all of the ingredients into your blender of choice (see our favorites, page 89) and blend, starting on the lowest setting and increasing power based on how smooth or chunky you'd like the results to be. We like to drink our smoothies right away, but you can keep them in an airtight container for up to 72 hours if you wish.

Feel free to play around with the ingredients as well as the amounts called for of each ingredient. There are no rules when it comes to making smoothies—so get creative!

MAKE YOUR OWN SMOOTHIE

Here are some of our favorite smoothie ingredients. Just choose a base liquid, add one to three building block ingredients, throw in a boost, and you're done.

BASE INGREDIENTS	BUILDING BLOCKS		BOOSTS	
Almond milk (or another nut milk)	Avocado	Papaya	Cacao	Lime
Coconut water	Banana	Peach	Cinnamon	Mint
Juice (apple, orange, and grapefruit are favorites)	Blueberries	Pear	E3Live	Parsley
Rice milk	Chard	Pineapple	Ginger	Spirulina
	Coconut	Romaine	Lemon	Turmeric
	Kale	Spinach		
	Mango	Strawberries		
	Orange	Watercress		

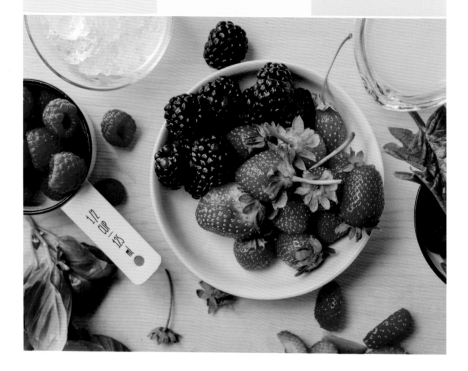

STRAWBERRY, BANANA, COCONUT, HERB

Strawberry banana is the vanilla milkshake of the smoothie world . . . add lemon, mint, and cilantro and take it to the next level.

MAKES ABOUT 1 (16-OUNCE) SERVING

2 bananas, peeled

1 cup strawberries

1 lemon, peeled

5 sprigs fresh mint

1 bunch fresh cilantro

1 cup coconut water

3 or 4 ice cubes

GOOD MORNING GREENS

Adding avocado makes this green smoothie a rich, delicious way to start your morning.

MAKES 1 TO 2 (16-OUNCE) SERVINGS

1 grapefruit, peeled (see box on page 66)

2 oranges, peeled

1 lime, peeled

1 cup orange juice

1 cup firmly packed spinach

½ head romaine

4 kale leaves

4 Swiss chard leaves

½ avocado, pitted and peeled

3 or 4 ice cubes

WATERMELON CHIA POWER SMOOTHIE

Cool watermelon, spicy ginger, and fresh mint combined are a great start for any smoothie; in this recipe, chia seeds add omega-3s and lower your blood pressure. Drink this one right away because the chia seeds will thicken the mixture as they sit in the liquid.

MAKES ABOUT 1 (16-OUNCE) SERVING

3 cups cubed watermelon

½-inch piece of fresh ginger, peeled and diced

5 fresh mint leaves

2 tablespoons chia seeds

1 cup firmly packed spinach

4 kale leaves

4 Swiss chard leaves

3 or 4 ice cubes

OUR FAVORITE BLENDERS

Vitamix and Blendtec are the holy grail of high-speed blenders—there are no other brands that can compete. Not only can you use these for smoothies, but also they are amazing for salad dressings, soups, and nut milks. The newest Vitamix motor is rated in horsepower, not watts, so you can imagine how quickly and efficiently it gets the job done. Both of these machines last forever, and starting around $400 each, they tend to be great investments. For slightly less impact on your wallet, try the Ninja Kitchen System or Breville's Hemisphere blender, which are both fantastic options and range from $99 to $200.

MANGO MINT

Sweet mango and fresh mint will make your mouth very happy.

MAKES ABOUT 1 (16-OUNCE) SERVING

1 mango, peeled and cubed

1 cup coconut water

1 cup firmly packed spinach

1 head romaine

1 bunch fresh mint

5 or 6 sprigs fresh parsley, to taste

3 or 4 ice cubes

BERRY BASIL BLISS

Basil with three kinds of berries makes for a sophisticated take on a smoothie.

MAKES ABOUT 1 (16-OUNCE) SERVING

½ cup raspberries

½ cup strawberries

½ cup blackberries

1 cup firmly packed spinach

5 fresh basil leaves

1 cup coconut water

3 or 4 ice cubes

MELON AND HERBS

Sweet cantaloupe and savory cilantro are an unexpected, but very welcome, pairing.

MAKES ABOUT 1 (16-OUNCE) SERVING

2 cups cubed cantaloupe

2 cups grapes

1 cup firmly packed spinach

1 small bunch fresh parsley

1 small bunch fresh cilantro

1 cup apple juice

3 or 4 ice cubes

TROPICAL GREENS

This is the kind of greens drink that goes really well with some sand, some sun, and the crash of waves. . . .

MAKES 1 TO 2 (16-OUNCE) SERVINGS

1 cup papaya

2 bananas, peeled

1 cup firmly packed spinach

3 Swiss chard leaves

1 cup coconut water

3 or 4 ice cubes

PEACHY GREENS

When peaches are in season, we rush to make this fruity green smoothie.

MAKES ABOUT 1 (16-OUNCE) SERVING

2 plums, pitted

1 peach, pitted

1 cucumber, peeled

1 head romaine

1 teaspoon pure vanilla extract

1 cup water or any nut milk

3 or 4 ice cubes

DANDELION BANANA DETOX

This is the kind of smoothie that makes people brag about how easy it is to detox.

MAKES ABOUT 1 (16-OUNCE) SERVING

2 pears, cored and chopped

1 banana, peeled

1 cup dandelion green leaves

1 cup firmly packed spinach

1 head romaine

1 cup apple juice

3 or 4 ice cubes

DAPHNE'S FAVORITE CHIA ALMOND SMOOTHIE

BY DAPHNE OZ

Daphne Oz is the cohost of ABC's hit show
The Chew *and author of the* New York Times
best-selling book Relish: An Adventure in Food,
Style, and Everyday Fun *and the national best
seller* The Dorm Room Diet. *Oz is a graduate
of the Institute for Integrative Nutrition and
received her culinary degree from the Natural
Gourmet Institute. She is also a dear friend
whom we turn to for creative recipe ideas that
make us look and feel great.*

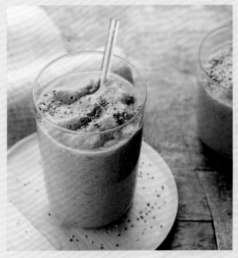

The fresh pineapple in this smoothie is the
real charmer; make sure you add at least a
few pieces of core to get maximum bromelain
(anti-inflammatory) benefits. Plus, the fresh
ginger is an immune- and energy-boosting
powerhouse. And then there's that dreamy
kale; it has so much fiber and is so easy to
slurp down in this delicious shake, to help
keep your waist whittled and your tummy
flat. This smoothie is rounded out with a little
almond butter for protein and fat, and it makes
a perfect meal any time of day.

Note: You can also empty your vitamin cap-
sules right into the blender or add cod liver oil
or flaxseed oil if that floats your boat!

MAKES ABOUT 1 (16-OUNCE) SERVING

¾ cup fresh pineapple chunks

1 cup firmly packed chopped kale

½ frozen banana, ¼ cup frozen mango
chunks, ½ avocado (pitted and peeled),
or ¼ cup yogurt (optional)

½- to 1-inch piece of fresh ginger, peeled
and grated, to taste

1 teaspoon almond butter

1 to 2 teaspoons chia seeds, to taste

1 cup juice, milk, almond milk, or water,
plus more as needed

3 or 4 ice cubes

Put all of the ingredients in a high-speed blender
and blend on high until smooth, adding more ice
or liquid as needed. Enjoy immediately because
the chia seeds will begin to thicken the mixture
as they sit in the liquid.

The following recipes were created by Justin Camilo, our director of operations. Justin knows his flavor profiles, and in addition to his juices, he is famous for making a mean smoothie. Our favorite days at the office are sampling days, when Justin walks around with yummy concoctions for us to try. Here are a few of those blends that we'd take over a piece of chocolate cake any day of the week.

COCONUT MINT CHIP

This smoothie tastes like mint chip ice cream. Seriously.

MAKES 1 TO 2 (16-OUNCE) SERVINGS

2 cups coconut water

½ avocado, pitted and peeled, or meat from 1 raw, young Thai coconut

5 fresh mint leaves

1 tablespoon cacao nibs

3 or 4 ice cubes

LIME IN THE COCONUT

Grab a beach umbrella and start sipping.

MAKES 1 TO 2 (12-OUNCE) SERVINGS

1 cup coconut water

Meat from 1 raw, young Thai coconut

½ avocado, pitted and peeled

1 banana, peeled

½ teaspoon spirulina powder

½ lime, peeled

3 or 4 ice cubes

TROPICAL GINGER

Rich and creamy with a tropical twist and warm notes of ginger, this is a staff favorite.

MAKES 1 TO 2 (12-OUNCE) SERVINGS

2 cups almond or rice milk

1 banana, peeled

1 cup papaya, cubed or coarsely chopped

1 peach, pitted

½-inch piece of fresh ginger, peeled

3 or 4 ice cubes

PEACHES AND CINNAMON

Creamy banana, summery fruit, and cinnamon make this a delicious treat at any time of day.

MAKES 1 TO 2 (16-OUNCE) SERVINGS

2 cups almond or rice milk

2 peaches, pitted

10 strawberries

1 banana, peeled

Pinch of cinnamon

3 or 4 ice cubes

ALMOND BUTTER CUP

This is luxurious enough to be served instead of dessert.

MAKES 1 TO 2 (12-OUNCE) SERVINGS

2 cups almond milk

1½ teaspoons raw cacao powder

1 banana, peeled

3 tablespoons raw almond butter

Pinch of cinnamon

3 or 4 ice cubes

COCONUT MINT CHIP

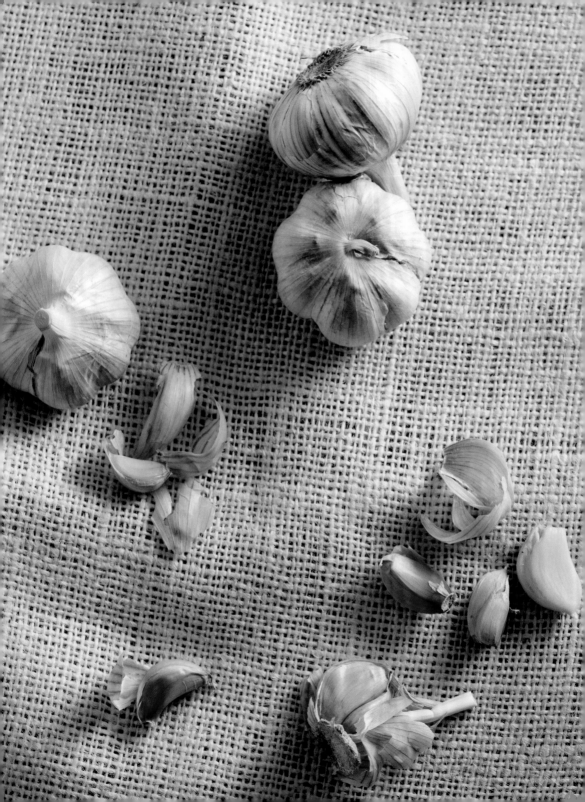

CHAPTER 9

SAVORY AND SPICY

Even green vegetables can start to taste sweet once you juice them. So for those days when we're in the mood for something different, we like to kick it up a notch with an added hint of garlic (yes, garlic!), cayenne pepper, and other savory ingredients. The recipes in this chapter have been created exclusively for those of you who prefer savory snacks over sweet ones, or dinner over dessert. Each of them can also be used to prepare a hot, tonic soup. Instead of juicing the ingredients listed, puree them in a high-speed blender, and then heat the mixture gently over a low flame.

We don't make any savory juices for our stores; we created these seven recipes exclusively for the book.

YES, GARLIC!

The most powerful compound in garlic is allicin, which is widely used in the alternative medicine field as an antibacterial, an antifungal, and a mechanism for promoting healthy cholesterol and blood pressure levels. Allicin has also been known to improve skin, even chronic acne, due to its unique ability to combat harmful pathogens and cleanse the gut. Finally, garlic is rich in the mineral sulfur, which is vital for blood sugar balance, detoxification, and the development of strong hair and nails. We use garlic in savory juices and a few of our elixir recipes—it's a great way to fight off seasonal colds. (Hold your nose while drinking if you have to—in a straight liquid form garlic is pretty potent, but it really does kick illness to the curb.)

BELL PEPPER, CARROTS, GREENS

Red bell peppers, which contain carotenoids and vitamin C, are a good choice if you crave a mild and sweet pepper flavor without the burning sensation brought on by chile peppers. Combined with carrots, this is a powerful immune booster.

MAKES 1 TO 2 (16-OUNCE) SERVINGS

3 carrots

1 large red bell pepper

Handful of spinach

3 or 4 collard green leaves, to taste

3 kale leaves

SPICY TOMATO, GREENS, FENNEL

This tomato-based juice might sound a little bit like a V8, but we guarantee that this one is better for you, better tasting, and more natural. While we don't recommend that you eat tomatoes if you're doing a cleanse, tomatoes do have a lot of health benefits. Rich in lycopene, a carotenoid pigment, tomatoes are also an excellent source of vitamin C and manganese. And in terms of phytonutrients, you can't do much better than tomatoes. They are incredibly antioxidant rich, which protects the cardiovascular system; they've been shown to regulate fat in the blood; and they are known for reducing the risk of heart disease. These are all great qualities for keeping your heart in tip-top shape.

MAKES 1 TO 2 (16-OUNCE) SERVINGS

2 large tomatoes

Handful of spinach

2 or 3 celery stalks, to taste

½ small fennel bulb, plus a few of the fronds

2 cloves garlic

½ teaspoon cayenne pepper

CABBAGE, CARROT, GARLIC, CELERY

Didn't your grandmother tell you to eat your cabbage? Ours did! And now we know why: cabbage is a powerful antioxidant, which helps with digestion and inflammation. When eaten raw (or in juice), cabbage can also lower cholesterol levels. We use both green and red cabbage in our recipes; try both and see which one you prefer.

MAKES 1 TO 2 (16-OUNCE) SERVINGS

5 carrots

¼ head red or green cabbage

1 or 2 cloves garlic, to taste

3 stalks celery

SPICY TOMATO, GREENS, FENNEL

GREENS WITH GARLIC AND LEMON

APPLE, LEMON, CUCUMBER, HERB

This is a light juice that has a sweet and savory balance; we love the use of herbs here. Herbs like basil and dill are some of the most under-appreciated superfoods in the plant family, often containing more nutrients than even their green vegetable counterparts and offering powerful detoxifying agents, too. We recommend trying different herbs in all of our juices to see what flavors work best for you.

MAKES 1 TO 2 (16-OUNCE) SERVINGS

1 large cucumber, peeled

3 fresh basil leaves

1 small bunch fresh dill

1 red or green apple

1 lemon, peeled

ROOTS WITH GARLIC, CUCUMBER, CELERY, AND LEMON

This has all the grounding of a roots juice (see chapter 4), with an extra spicy kick.

MAKES 1 TO 2 (16-OUNCE) SERVINGS

3 carrots

½ beet (see box on page 54)

1 clove garlic

½ lemon, peeled

½ cucumber, peeled

3 celery stalks

TOMATO, CARROT, RADISH, LEMON

Radishes are known to have a natural cooling effect on the body—their clean, spicy flavor and high water content are perfect in the warmer months. Adding lemon here gives you a double dose of vitamin C.

MAKES 1 TO 2 (16-OUNCE) SERVINGS

3 or 4 medium tomatoes, to taste

3 carrots

4 radishes, leaves and stems removed

1 lemon, peeled

GREENS WITH GARLIC AND LEMON

Chard is extremely high in vitamins K, A, and C, as well as an important source of the minerals magnesium, manganese, potassium, and iron. Its ability to support not only the cardiovascular system but also the bones and muscles makes chard an athlete-friendly vegetable. Chard leaves are very large, so you get a lot of bang for your buck when juicing as compared to other leafy greens, which require a lot of leaves to get a good amount of juice.

MAKES 1 TO 2 (8-OUNCE) SERVINGS

5 or 6 rainbow chard leaves, to taste

A few leaves of cabbage

4 celery stalks

1 clove garlic

½ cucumber, peeled

½ lemon, peeled

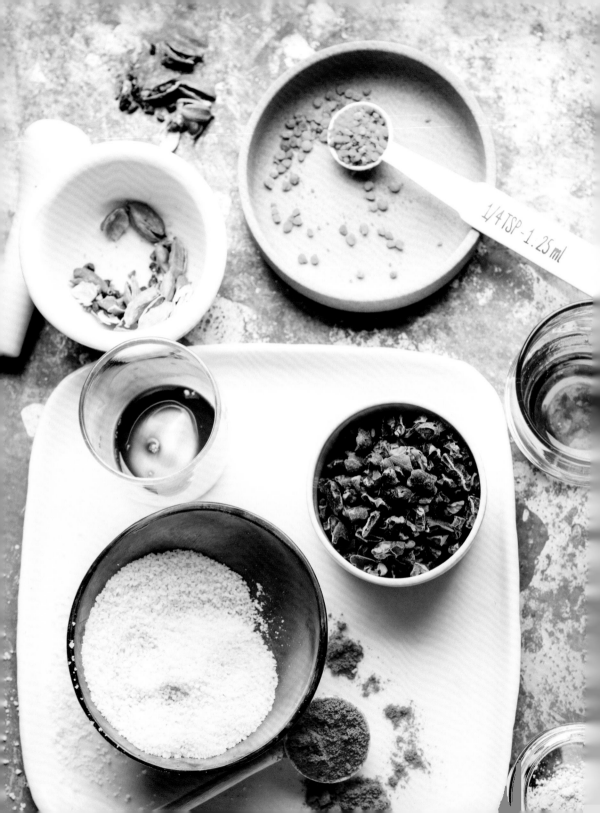

CHAPTER 10

ELIXIRS AND FLAVORED WATERS

As our bodies naturally get cleaner and juice and smoothies become a regular part of our diets, it's amazing how much we crave natural alternatives to other beverages. Our elixirs are usually taken as shots and are designed to alleviate symptoms of discomfort, from the common cold to a sour stomach.

We created our flavored waters in response to the shelves and shelves of sugary "waters" found in every grocery store. It might seem as if those waters are healthy, but in reality, dye and sugars have been added to most of them, and the ones that are sugar-free are also filled with chemicals.

One of the most important factors in good health—one that we can't stress enough—is staying hydrated. We are mostly made up of water. It is a vital resource for our bodies and our survival depends on it. But drinking sugar water that is assumed to have added vitamins is very different from drinking the pure, high-quality water that we're talking about.

Water has different levels of quality, which is why it's important to drink filtered water. We absolutely love alkaline water filters; however, these are quite expensive and we know that most people cannot afford to invest in this equipment at home. Instead, just make sure you are drinking at least eight glasses per day of the best filtered water you can get your hands on. If it has a very high pH (above 8.5), all the better.

It can sometimes feel as though drinking all that plain water is a chore. While it's refreshing, it can lack the vibrancy or flavor of those store-bought waters if that's what you're used to drinking. To make water a little more interesting, we created flavored waters, including our Chlorophyll H_2O (page 138) and our Aloe Vera H_2O (page 137). However, you can also add many other ingredients to water that not only have health benefits but also taste more interesting.

We like to call these flavored water combinations our version of spa water, that delicious water you drink while waiting for a massage to begin. So sit back, relax, and sip—your body will thank you. And if you're feeling creative, make up your own mixes—you can't go wrong. All of the water recipes can be stored in the refrigerator for up to three days.

While we do not make any medical claims, we do know that our elixirs and flavored waters contain natural, whole-foods ingredients that have been used to help people for thousands of years. We are not reinventing the wheel here—we're just making it easy for you to create these healing drinks for yourself at home.

The recipes in this chapter can be used as precleanse and postcleanse additions, or when you simply want to kick up your immune system a notch. Combined in different ways, these ingredients are known to aid in a multitude of ailments. Most of these recipes are super simple to make and use ingredients that have already been mentioned in "Stocking Your Juice Pantry" (page 24) or used in other juicing recipes. So get ready to toss back a shot or pour yourself a flavored water chaser; you're on your way to feeling good.

GET ESSENTIAL

Another way to get concentrated benefits from and flavor into your water is to use essential oils. Essential oils are natural aromatic compounds found in the seeds, bark, stems, roots, flowers, and other parts of plants. They are used for a wide range of applications to improve emotional and physical wellness.

Our favorite brands are dōTERRA and Young Living, and we can't rave about them enough. The quality of these brands is so high that many of the oils can actually be ingested (oils of lesser quality can usually be used only topically). Some of our favorite essential oils are lemon, ginger, grapefruit, lavender, peppermint, and oregano. Add a couple of drops to water, and it gives your senses such a buzz. When you imagine how calming it is to smell lavender, just think about what it feels like to drink it!

But seriously, each essential oil serves a purpose. You get a more intense and concentrated flavor experience with lemon oil, for example, than you would by squeezing a lemon into water because you are also getting powerful antioxidants from the rind, a portion of the lemon that is usually removed before juicing and rarely eaten aside from lemon zest.

COLD-AND-FLU ELIXIR

If you already feel the tingle of sickness in your throat and your nose is starting to run, or if you just want to kick your immunity into high gear, try this remedy. It is even more intense than the Immunity Elixir (page 104) and it stings a bit going down, but we're telling you, it does the trick. Make sure you buy wild Mediterranean oregano oil, which can be found online or at most natural foods stores (see the Resources, page 144). We can feel it fighting off the cold as soon as we take a shot of this stuff. Even on its own, oil of oregano is a powerful force against bacteria, so in combination with lemon, flaxseed oil, ginger, and cayenne, it's likely to produce results quickly. Mix everything together and take it as a shot.

MAKES ABOUT 1 (3-OUNCE) SHOT

10 drops oil of oregano

¼ cup flaxseed oil

1 tablespoon fresh ginger juice

½ lemon, juiced by hand or in a juicer

Pinch of cayenne pepper (optional)

ALKALINITY ELIXIR

This was inspired by our Morning Alkalizer (page 138), which is great for balancing your pH (see page 14). The addition of garlic here adds an immunity boost as well. We like this elixir because you can make it once a week. Blend all the ingredients together in your blender and store it in an airtight container in the refrigerator for up to 1 week. To use it, combine 1 tablespoon of the elixir with ½ cup of water (or juice) and drink it down. Add a squeeze of lemon if you'd like. You can also mix 1 tablespoon of the elixir with extra-virgin olive oil and lemon juice for a tangy, unprocessed salad dressing!

MAKES ABOUT 16 (0.5-OUNCE) SERVINGS

3 cloves garlic, peeled

½ cup manuka honey

½ cup apple cider vinegar

SOUR STOMACH ELIXIR

We love basil in our salads and on pizza, but most people don't know that it also soothes indigestion and can alleviate acid reflux. We add raw honey to alkalize, but you could also add lemon here or keep it super simple and take this with just the herbs and water. Steep the basil leaves in the warm water for 5 minutes, stir in the honey, and sip slowly.

MAKES ABOUT 1 (8-OUNCE) SERVING

Small handful of fresh basil leaves

1 cup warm water

1 tablespoon manuka honey

INFLAMMATION ELIXIR

We take this on a regular basis as a preventative measure against disease and discomfort. We find it to be a natural pain reliever and helpful in reducing redness in the skin. Add raw honey for a touch of sweetness. Combine everything together and drink it warm like tea.

MAKES ABOUT 1 (8-OUNCE) SERVING

1 cup warm water

¼ teaspoon ground turmeric or grated fresh turmeric

½ lemon, juiced by hand or in a juicer

IMMUNITY ELIXIR

This isn't the easiest elixir to stomach at first, but nothing beats a shot of this potent combination during cold-and-flu season to boost your immune system. It also keeps digestion regular. We like to chase this with a cup of Citrus 5 (page 67) for an added boost. This is also a great supplement for a cleanse. Mix everything together and take it as a shot.

MAKES ABOUT 1 (2-OUNCE) SHOT

1 tablespoon extra-virgin olive oil

1 large clove garlic, juiced or minced

½ lemon, juiced by hand or in a juicer

1 tablespoon fresh ginger juice, or 1 teaspoon finely minced fresh ginger

Pinch of cayenne pepper

METABOLISM ELIXIR

We drink this to rev up our metabolisms and stave off cravings. It also aids in digestion and just feels good for the system. Stir everything together and let the flavor of the cinnamon stick settle into the water.

MAKES ABOUT 1 (8-OUNCE) SERVING

1 cup water

Pinch of cayenne pepper

1 cinnamon stick

½ lemon, juiced by hand or in a juicer

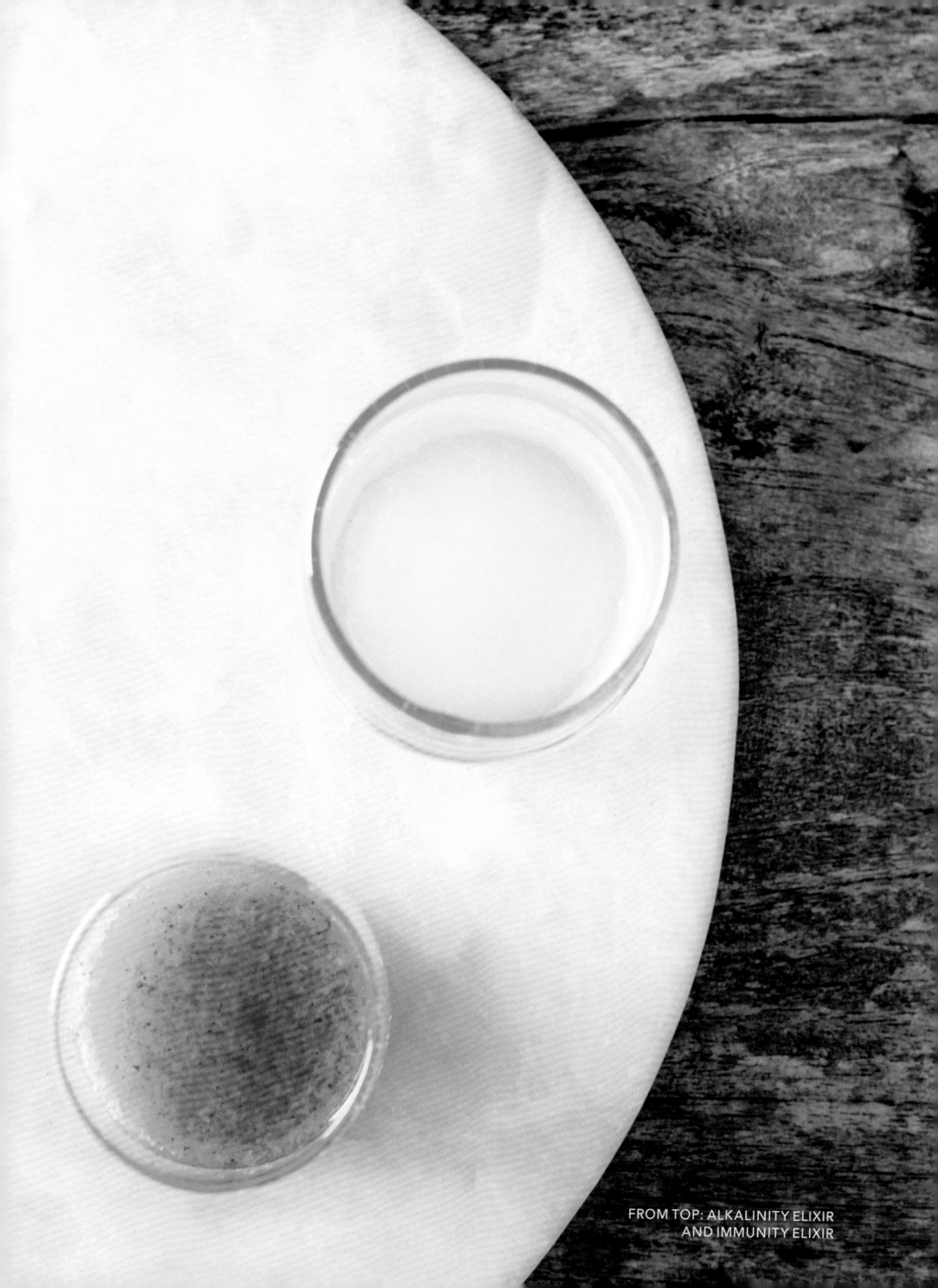

FROM TOP: ALKALINITY ELIXIR
AND IMMUNITY ELIXIR

BLACKBERRY SAGE WATER

Combine all of the
ingredients, muddling
the blackberries and sage
into the water. Allow the
mixture to steep for at
least 45 minutes before
drinking.

**MAKES 2 (16-OUNCE)
SERVINGS**

2 large sprigs sage
1 cup blackberries
4 cups water

LEMON GINGER MINT WATER

Crush the ginger and mint together with a mortar and pestle or a fork. Combine with the water and lemon slices and allow the mixture to steep for at least 45 minutes before drinking.

MAKES 2 (16-OUNCE) SERVINGS

3-inch piece of fresh ginger, peeled

5 sprigs fresh mint

4 cups water

½ lemon, sliced

CITRUS WATER

Combine all of the ingredients and allow the mixture to steep for at least 45 minutes before drinking.

MAKES 2 (16-OUNCE) SERVINGS

2 lemons, thinly sliced

½ grapefruit, thinly sliced

1 orange, thinly sliced

4 cups water

CUCUMBER BASIL WATER

Combine all of the ingredients, crushing the basil a little to release its flavors. Allow the mixture to steep for at least 45 minutes before drinking. This recipe is also great with some thin slices of lemon for an additional alkaline boost.

MAKES 2 (16-OUNCE) SERVINGS

3 cucumbers, thinly sliced

Small handful of fresh basil leaves

1 lemon, thinly sliced (optional)

4 cups water

KIWI-CUCUMBER FACE MASK WITH HONEY AND AVOCADO

A diet rich in fruits and vegetables can help you achieve glowing skin from the inside out. You can also apply some produce directly to the skin to reap the benefits. The hydrating skin mask below gives you another way to use up the fruit and veggie pulp you create when juicing.

Kiwi and cucumber are both antioxidant rich and incredibly hydrating. As Dr. Lancer mentioned (see page 28), kiwi contains vitamins C and E, which promote collagen production in the skin. This mask also includes honey and avocado, whose oils, vitamins, and mineral content make a wonderful natural skin moisturizer.

MAKES ABOUT 1½ CUPS

2 kiwis, peeled

2 small cucumbers, peeled

1 tablespoon raw honey

½ avocado, pitted and peeled

In your juicer, juice the kiwis and cucumbers and reserve the juice to drink (yum!). Remove the pulp from the juicer and place it in a mixing bowl. Add the honey and avocado and mash everything together until creamy.

Apply the mask to your face, avoiding the eyes and mouth area, and leave it on for 15 to 20 minutes. To remove the mask, wash it off gently with warm water. Enjoy your glow!

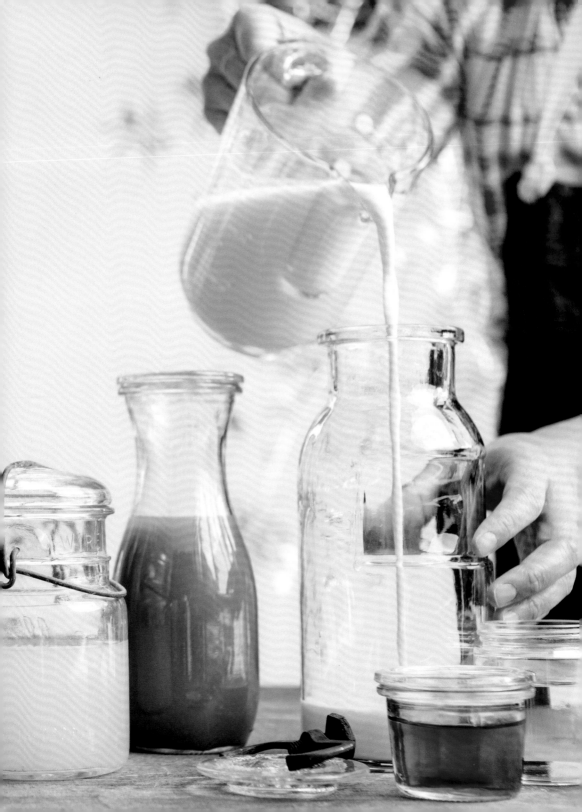

CLEANSING

Cleansing has become a hot topic lately—but it's not a modern invention. People have been using diets and fasting for spiritual, religious, and health reasons for centuries. When we talk about cleansing, we don't mean fasting or starvation. We literally mean *cleaning up your act*. Cleansing to us is not about deprivation but about getting clean, giving ourselves maximum nutrition from whole, wholesome fruits and vegetables, and reducing our dependence on processed foods that are at the root of so many health crises.

Adding juice to your diet is a way of boosting nutrition and getting back to healthy basics. Cleansing is about taking that clean eating approach a step further, giving your system a break, and giving you a chance to tune into your body.

Periodic cleanses can really do incredible and positive work for your digestive system, and in turn, it creates a ripple effect that is evident in all areas of your health and life, including the mental and emotional aspects. It may take a concerted effort on your part, but once you begin to feel the benefits, you understand why it is so worth it.

resting promotes healing

For most of us, with our hectic schedules, vacations are few and far between. But when we do indulge in them, we usually find that our ability to go with the flow improves, and we operate with a clearer and lighter sense of being. On vacation, we nourish our human need to unwind.

Your digestive system is similar. It spends all of its time working hard for you, taking everything you ingest and breaking it down in an effort to effectively distribute nutrients and discard waste. The more you eat, the harder it works. And if you are eating processed foods, foods that have the nutrients removed, your body works even harder with no payoff except sluggishness and potentially harsher consequences like diabetes and obesity and heart disease.

why we need to push reset

The reality is that we live in a polluted world. Toxins and chemicals abound in everything from the food we eat and the makeup and clothes we wear to the air we breathe. It's shocking how many of these toxins penetrate our bodily systems and affect us on many levels, both physical and mental.

This toxic pollution has been linked to diseases like cancer, as well as a plethora of chronic illnesses, such as irritable bowel syndrome, joint disorders, migraine headaches, and depression, to name a few. We can work to clean up our planet, but we can also pay attention to what we put into our bodies. Even if you eat a relatively healthy diet and

you exercise regularly, this maintenance is not necessarily enough to repair your entire system and flush out the toxins that are hiding in your cells, tissues, and organs. That's where detoxification and cleansing come in.

When you cleanse, you are replacing meals full of processed foods and junk with clean, healthy foods. Cleansing is essentially composed of the following:

- Putting clean foods in
- Eliminating what is not clean

Now, think about what it would do for your health to be able to give your digestive system a well-deserved *break* from all of its hard work, a chance to take a vacation from the stress that it bears on a regular basis, and a chance to clean up its act, refresh, and reboot. Your body (and soul) would most likely thrive given this opportunity. That's what cleansing is: a way of hitting the reset button.

And it doesn't have to be extreme. Over the next two chapters, you'll learn how to ease into (and out of) a cleanse, and how to take care of yourself while cleansing. You'll also get suggestions on how to incorporate the cleansing effects of juice into your daily schedule, even if you want to keep eating breakfast.

Because for us, cleansing isn't about imposing a rigid structure. It's about welcoming new ideas, supporting our health, and taking care of ourselves from the inside out.

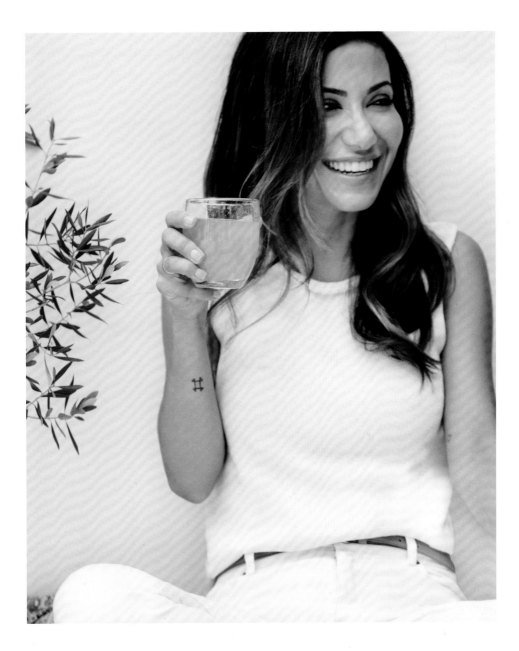

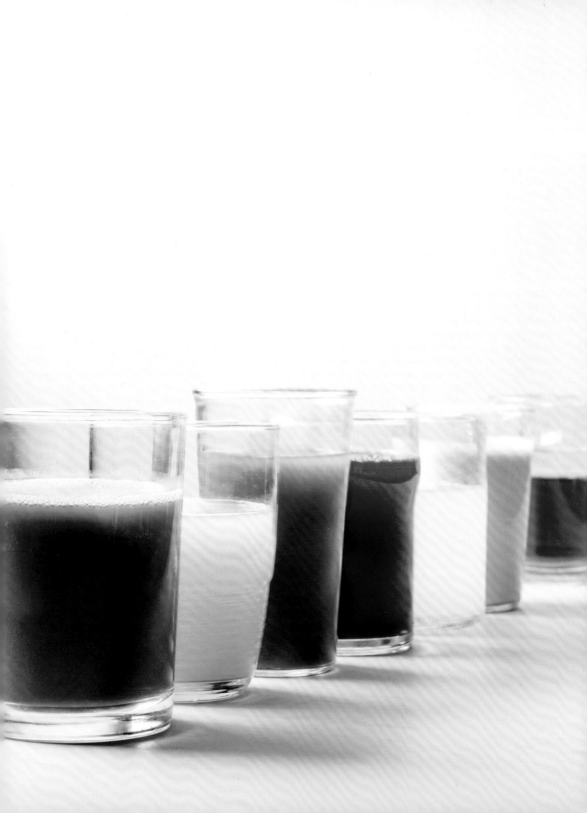

CHAPTER 11

CHOOSING AND PREPARING FOR YOUR CLEANSE

There are many ways to cleanse. When we first encountered it as a practice, one of our hesitations was how rigid so many of the experts were when it came to this style of cleansing or that. In our case, we're not experts; we're users. We're juicers. We have personally experienced how amazing we felt after doing a juice cleanse that was suited to our particular needs and styles. And that's what we want for you: to experience the astounding effects that juicing can have on your life and your general sense of well-being.

What we found was that cleansing removes the "noise" inside our bodies and allows us to *hear* that voice that tells us what it needs. Listening is the miraculous step that comes next, where we actually take this information and use it to make choices.

Our approach to cleansing is never about preaching or dogma or fasting or starving or dieting or self-deprivation. It is about awareness, consciousness, and focus; about being

aware of what we put into our bodies; about listening to our bodies, a great gift we can give ourselves that society doesn't always support; about taking the time to shift out of the paradigm that we are currently living in and creating a new truth. And most of all, it's about nourishing ourselves—by removing what is bad through detoxification and giving our bodies and minds the power of nutritionally dense foods, which leads to clarity and balance.

getting started: precleansing

Now that you're ready to start drinking your fruits and vegetables in the most beneficial way possible, there are a number of ways that you can get started. We have classic menus that you can follow, or you can customize your cleanse by taking an à la carte approach. The more you juice, the more you get comfortable blending and mixing, the more you will find yourself expanding your recipe repertoire.

This might sound a little odd, but before you cleanse, you need to precleanse. You've got to get your body ready for the experience that is coming, and that involves cleaning out your system as much as possible *before* you start your official cleanse. The cleaner you are to begin with, the more prepared you will be for an all-liquid diet. You'll experience fewer side effects, and you'll be better able to reap the benefits of the cleanse and sustain your new positive habits once you finish your cleanse. In the same way, after your cleanse, you'll want to ease back into a regular diet, instead of slamming your body from its restful, healing phase back into the intensity of seven-course meals or even soup-salad-sandwich.

The best way to prepare for a juice cleanse is to follow what is called an elimination diet for a few days prior to the cleanse. This removes all of the inflammatory and processed foods from your diet (see the box below). Following an elimination diet can be an incredibly healing way to eat. According to Dr. Alejandro Junger (see page 12), eliminating certain foods from our diets can change the state of our health and well-being (read more about this in his amazing books, *Clean* and *Clean Gut*, or on his website, www.cleanprogram.com). Basically, when you consistently eat foods that you are allergic to or that are hard to digest, your body's immune response kicks in to defend you. And you already know that inflammation in the body can cause disease. Dr. Junger recommends that people enjoy a diet mostly consisting of organic vegetables, brown rice, beans, fish, lean protein, fruits, and nuts because this way of eating can alleviate many common symptoms of inflammation.

ELIMINATE THESE FOODS FROM YOUR PRECLEANSE DIET

If it comes from a box and has more than one ingredient, you really want to avoid it. Processed food can be very difficult for our bodies to break down, and even the healthy-looking products we see in the market aren't as healthy as they might at first seem.

Alcohol	Cow's milk (goat's milk is okay, but limit your consumption)	Eggs	Red meat (or other nonorganic meat)
Caffeine		Gluten	Shellfish
Corn		Nightshade veggies (see box on page 115)	White sugar

It's also important to avoid processed soy products. Look for the words *soy protein isolate* on the label. This is what you want to avoid. Soy protein isolate can be found in various soy ice creams, protein powders, energy bars, and many other food items.

You can't expect your body to understand what is going on when one day you are eating a carne asado taco with the works and suddenly the next day you are drinking only green juice! It's simply confusing for your system and, ultimately, counterproductive. Eliminating processed and inflammatory foods from your diet a few days before starting a cleanse allows you to ingest large amounts of juice without shocking your body. The foods you can trust are the foods that are simple and most natural. We are talking mostly fruits and vegetables, and a moderate amount of the cleanest and healthiest versions of grains and lean meats and fish.

Because it's not always easy to figure out how to cook clean and healthy food, we collaborated with one of our favorite chefs, Pamela Salzman, to create a few recipes for breakfast, lunch, and dinner that will get you engaged in the kitchen and inspired to keep eating unprocessed, nutrient-dense meals (see page 137). We met Pamela at a local cooking class and instantly fell in love with her no-nonsense approach to preparing healthy foods that taste incredible. Cooking can be easier than you ever imagined—and it can also be really fun, too!

Try one or all of these recipes during the three days just prior to starting your cleanse. You can also enjoy any of these recipes as you are easing out of your cleanse. If you're prone to improvisation when it comes to menu planning, use these recipes as suggestions and change them up as you like, or go completely off the menu if you already have healthy options that are elimination diet–friendly.

BREAKFAST

- Warm Coconut Millet Porridge (page 140)

- Painted Fruit (page 143)

LUNCH

- Big Green Detox Salad (page 137)

- Warm Quinoa and Vegetable Salad (page 142)

- Lentil Dal (page 141)

DINNER

- Halibut in Parchment with Zucchini, Fennel, and Capers (page 142)

- Cauliflower Tabbouleh (page 141)

- Spring Green Minestrone (page 140)

LET'S TALK ABOUT NIGHTSHADES

Nightshades refer to a group of vegetables, including tomatoes, eggplant, sweet and hot peppers, paprika, and potatoes, that may cause a food sensitivity in some individuals. Nightshades contain compounds called alkaloids, which are believed to cause adverse symptoms in some people, especially those who suffer from chronic inflammation, joint pain, and nerve conditions. You'll find tomatoes in some of our savory juices; and while not everyone is affected by this food group, we like to eliminate nightshades while cleansing, just to be sure.

Once you experience the benefits of an elimination diet, if you really give it a solid go, you might not want to go back to your previous eating habits. That's the power of results. And that's why all those healthy eaters and juicers are doing it: not because it hurts, but because they begin to feel such incredible changes that they can't even remember craving junk food to begin with. And ultimately, it resets your patterns and brings you back down to what you truly need.

For now, you've been eating your quinoa and your kale salads, your spinach and brown rice and chickpea dinners. Good for you! Now you are ready to start your juice cleanse.

choosing the best cleanse for you

While we promote both three- and five-day cleanses at Pressed Juicery, we don't push a strict regimen to achieve a certain level of health. We believe that every individual is different and what works for one person may not work for you. There are many different paths to healthy eating and lifestyle habits; try out the different options we describe below and feel how your body and mind react to the choices.

Never aim to do more than you think your body can handle—again, this is not about starvation or deprivation, and it is certainly not a race. As long as you are doing your best to eat well most of the time—based on a proper pH balance and eliminating toxins and foods that trigger sensitivity—you are on the right track. This is about being better

in little ways that add up and tailoring your habits to the bio-individuality that makes up who you are.

You don't necessarily have to do a full-blown cleanse to integrate juicing into your diet. We're all at different levels, and we want to meet you in the middle. If you *want* to do a cleanse, that's great; we include our most popular ones here. But you can also ease into juicing: try it out, see how you like the taste of the juices, and pay attention to how your body feels.

On the following pages, we've listed a few simple ways to start juicing regularly, followed by our suggestions and guidelines for a classic cleanse. Choose what makes sense for you today, and change up your approach two weeks down the line if you feel you want to scale up or down. After a couple of weeks of drinking a juice every morning, you might decide you want to do a three-day cleanse. Or, if that sounds too intense, try a one-day juice cleanse. There's a ton of flexibility here; we just want you to drink juice, plain and simple.

DRINK ONE JUICE OR BLENDED DRINK PER DAY

We'd like to invite you to start every day with a green juice, even if you are also going to eat breakfast. This behavior adds up and can make a huge difference to your colon and overall health. This isn't a meal replacement; it's just added nutrition. Soon you'll begin to crave healthier foods. Try to make it your mission to include one green juice every day of

A WORD ON GMOS

BY LAUREN FELTS, IN-HOUSE NUTRITIONIST AT PRESSED JUICERY

GMO stands for *genetically modified organism*, which is a plant or animal that has been created by altering its genes. *GMO* is a term that is now well-known within the health industry, but what does it mean exactly? With GMOs, genes are taken from various sources and combined to obtain a certain desired trait or characteristic. For instance, corn is one of the most common foods that is genetically modified, and that is because Americans love corn that is sweet, juicy, and large in size. It is in a corn farmer's interest to grow lots of corn that is sweet, juicy, and large. As a result, corn has been modified to carry these traits as well as to be resistant against the pesky bugs that oftentimes attack it.

The problem with genetically modified foods is that nature is not a closed system, and therefore these GMO species easily cross-pollinate into other areas, contaminating our entire ecosystem. This becomes a problem since it becomes more difficult to identify GMO and non-GMO foods.

So how do GMOs impact our health? The research into GMOs is still incomplete, with many answers in regard to their health effects still left unanswered. But there have been a multitude of studies done on animals indicating that GMOs may cause a wide range of health effects, such as "potentially precancerous cell growth, damaged immune systems, smaller brains, livers, and testicles, partial atrophy or increased density of the liver, odd-shaped cell nuclei and other unexplained anomalies, false pregnancies and higher death rates" (American Academy of Environmental Medicine). Therefore, we believe that it is extremely important to avoid consuming any food that has been genetically modified, to help prevent the occurrence of any disease or condition long term.

the week, the way you would drink coffee (or instead of your morning coffee!).

You can also replace one meal per day with a blended smoothie (see chapter 8) or savory soup (see page 139). Drinking blended, nutritious foods also gives your digestion a rest because your body doesn't have to work so hard to break down the food; the blender has already done some of the work for you. Add ingredients that give you the protein you need (like almonds, chia seeds, or plant-based protein powder), but don't add dairy or extra salt or sugar.

DRINK ONLY JUICE UNTIL DINNER

Half of us forget to eat when we're busy and going about our normal routines. But there is nothing worse than going all day without eating, because it often leads to bingeing; you end up being so desperate for food that you'll eat just about anything.

If you're not yet ready to tackle an all-liquid cleanse, drinking juice all day until dinner is a great way to get your nutrition easily and give your body a rest, but still get the extra fuel at dinnertime. You can do this as often as you'd like, and making a habit of it (every two weeks, for instance) makes it more likely that you'll stick to eating well in between. As your body adjusts to drinking juice regularly, over time you'll start to crave healthier foods as the toxins make their way out.

Drink at least four vegetable-based juices during the day and eat one item from our pre- and postcleanse recipe section (see pages 137 to 143) in the evening.

DRINK ONLY LIQUIDS ONCE PER WEEK

With this approach, you choose one day per week when you're going to get all of your nutrition in liquid form: through juices, smoothies, blended soups, elixirs, and so on. The rest of the week, you eat normally, meaning healthily, of course. This is one of our favorite ways to drink juice because it allows us to cleanse in a very manageable way. And of course, you can tailor this approach to your needs and do it once every two weeks or once a month.

Here's what our one-day menu looks like:

- Morning Alkalizer (page 138)
- Green juice (for breakfast; see chapter 3)
- Green juice (for a snack)
- Green juice (for a snack)
- Smoothie (for lunch; see chapter 8)
- Citrus juice (for a snack; see chapter 5)
- Our Favorite Blended Soup (for dinner; page 139)
- Aloe Vera H_2O (page 137) or 1 tablespoon of extra-virgin olive oil before bed

GET ORGANIZED FOR YOUR CLEANSE

Although cleansing at home takes extra effort, here are some tips to help you get organized for your cleanse.

- Clear out your fridge so you have room to store all of your produce.

- Choose your cleanse menu, make a list of all the ingredients you'll need, and shop accordingly. To save time, choose one greens, one citrus, and one roots recipe per day.

- Prep your produce ahead of time and store it in resealable bags or glass containers. When you are ready to make your juice, just pop the ingredients in the juicer.

- Make a large batch of any water-based drink, like Aloe Vera H_2O (page 137), Chlorophyll H_2O (page 138), Citrus 1 (page 64), or flavored waters (pages 106–7), and store them in the refrigerator.

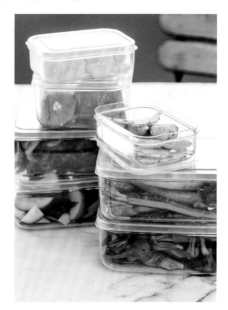

- Make a large batch of almond milk (see chapter 7) and store it in the refrigerator. If you choose a smoothie or soup, you can also do the prep at the beginning of the cleanse and make a large batch.

- Double or triple the juice recipes and portion them out into containers for simplified transport. Take them with you in a cooler bag or store them in the fridge until you're ready to drink them. (Note: This method will oxidize the juices faster. Generally, we recommend making vegetable-based juices right before you consume them to get the most nutrients during your cleanse.)

THE CLASSIC CLEANSE

If you're an expert cleanser, you know what to expect and how your body reacts when you cleanse. If this is your first time, we advise that you go slow and start with the cleanse that has the highest calorie content (Cleanse 1), adding more roots juices and a soup or smoothie for your final liquid of the day. Drink five or six (8- to 16-ounce) juices a day. We want you to get the maximum nutrient content and calories. Once you've acclimated and gotten a feel for what cleansing feels like, you can up the ante on your next go-round.

One thing we do recommend is making sure that the fruit and vegetable scales tip toward the vegetables. We add fruit to many of our juices and encourage people to drink them in moderation, but while cleansing, it is recommended that the majority of produce you juice be from the vegetable kingdom. Lucky for you, we have a lot of really great veggie-based recipes that will please your palate and help you get the most out of your cleanse. You can experiment and do this any way you like, but the more green juices and less sugar, the more intense the level of cleansing and the less calories. At the same time, you must know that cleansing is not a means by which to starve yourself. When you do a juice cleanse, you should be consuming maximum amounts of nutrition, just not in solid form.

We also recommend that you drink an almond milk or cashew milk as part of any cleanse. Since not all of us can eat nuts (because it's a common allergy these days), if you would like to forgo almond milk or cashew milk in place of something else, we recommend one of our smoothies (see chapter 8).

And remember: Always consult your doctor before beginning a cleanse.

SCHEDULE

- **Wake-up:** Morning Alkalizer (page 138)
- **Breakfast:** Green juice (see chapter 3)
- **Snack:** Citrus juice (see chapter 5)
- **Lunch:** Green juice
- **Snack:** Green, citrus, or roots (see chapter 4) juice
- **Dinner:** Green, citrus, or roots juice
- **Snack:** Almond milk (see chapter 7), The Best Veggie Broth (page 139), or Our Favorite Blended Soup (page 139)
- **Before bed:** Aloe Vera H_2O (page 137)
- **Note:** Drink at least 16 ounces of Chlorophyll H_2O (page 138) throughout the day. Some people also like to add an extra almond milk to this program.

CLEANSE 1

This is recommended for beginners and anyone who prefers to have extra calories, such as athletes. We created this program as an introduction to the world of cleansing. The juice selection is richer, heavier, and a bit more caloric than the other cleanses, resulting in a gentler cleanse. It is designed for the majority of people out there who know they can improve their diet and are ready to get on track. We find that our customers feel this is the easiest plan to stick to, as it usually keeps them pretty full.

SCHEDULE

- **Wake-up:** Morning Alkalizer (page 138)
- **Breakfast:** Green juice (see chapter 3)
- **Snack:** Roots juice (see chapter 4)
- **Lunch:** Green juice
- **Snack:** Citrus juice (see chapter 5)
- **Dinner:** Roots juice
- **Snack:** Almond milk (see chapter 7), The Best Veggie Broth (page 139), or Our Favorite Blended Soup (page 139)
- **Before bed:** Aloe Vera H_2O (page 137)
- **Note:** Drink at least 16 ounces of Chlorophyll H_2O (page 138) throughout the day. Some people also like to add an extra almond milk to this program.

CLEANSE 2

This is our most popular juice cleanse. We recommend Cleanse 2 to those who are more experienced with eating mostly whole, unprocessed foods and who have even tried cleansing before. It is perfect for those who would like a deep cleanse but are not quite ready to drink all greens all day long.

SCHEDULE

- **Wake-up:** Morning Alkalizer (page 138)
- **Breakfast:** Green juice (see chapter 3)
- **Snack:** Citrus juice (see chapter 5)
- **Lunch:** Roots juice (see chapter 4)
- **Snack:** Citrus juice
- **Dinner:** Green juice
- **Snack:** Almond milk (see chapter 7), The Best Veggie Broth (page 139), or Our Favorite Blended Soup (page 139)
- **Before bed:** Aloe Vera H_2O (page 137)
- **Note:** Drink at least 16 ounces of Chlorophyll H_2O (page 138) throughout the day.

CLEANSE 3

This is for the green juice lovers. This cleanse is the lightest that we offer. It tends to have fewer calories and sugar than Cleanses 1 and 2, so it is not for the faint of heart. We recommend Cleanse 3 only to experienced cleansers who are comfortable with the regimen and who have been maintaining a clean diet for at least six months.

SCHEDULE

- **Wake-up:** Morning Alkalizer (page 138)
- **Breakfast:** Green juice (see chapter 3)
- **Snack:** Citrus juice (see chapter 5)
- **Lunch:** Green juice
- **Snack:** Green juice
- **Dinner:** Green juice
- **Snack:** Almond milk (see chapter 7), The Best Veggie Broth (page 139), or Our Favorite Blended Soup (page 139)
- **Before bed:** Aloe Vera H$_2$0 (page 137)
- **Note:** Drink at least 16 ounces of Chlorophyll H$_2$0 (page 138) throughout the day.

SUPPLEMENT WITH ELIXIRS

We highly recommend adding a shot of Immunity Elixir (page 104), Cold-and-Flu Elixir (page 103), or Alkalinity Elixir (page 103) for an extra boost while cleansing. The garlic and lemon will kick your immune system into gear, while the ginger helps digestion, the vinegar alkalizes, and the flaxseed and olive oils aid in elimination.

nourish yourself

Eating clean, healthy food is much larger than losing weight and preventing illness. It is about cleansing all areas of our spiritual, emotional, and physical beings and becoming balanced and truly happy. It sounds crazy to some, but what we feed ourselves is not relegated purely to what is on our plate—we need to nourish our souls as well. But it is all connected; holistic transformation is possible, and the first step is changing the way we look at the framework of health altogether—being able to understand that we are capable and worthy of flourishing health, inner peace, and true joy.

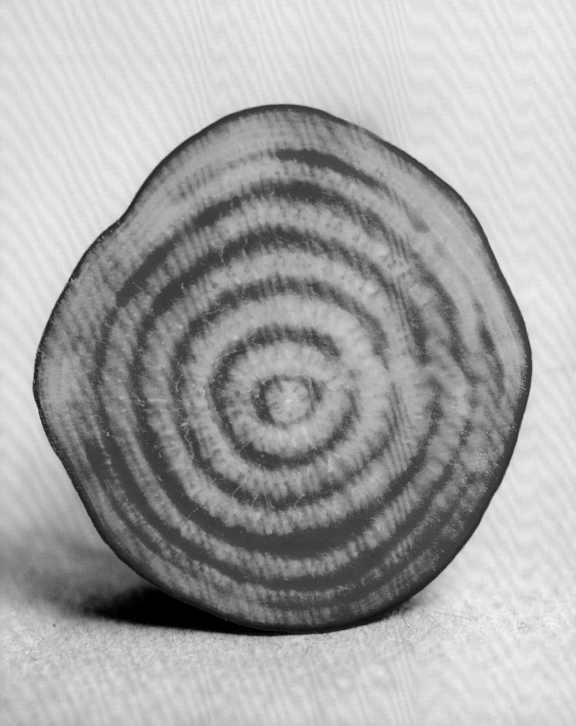

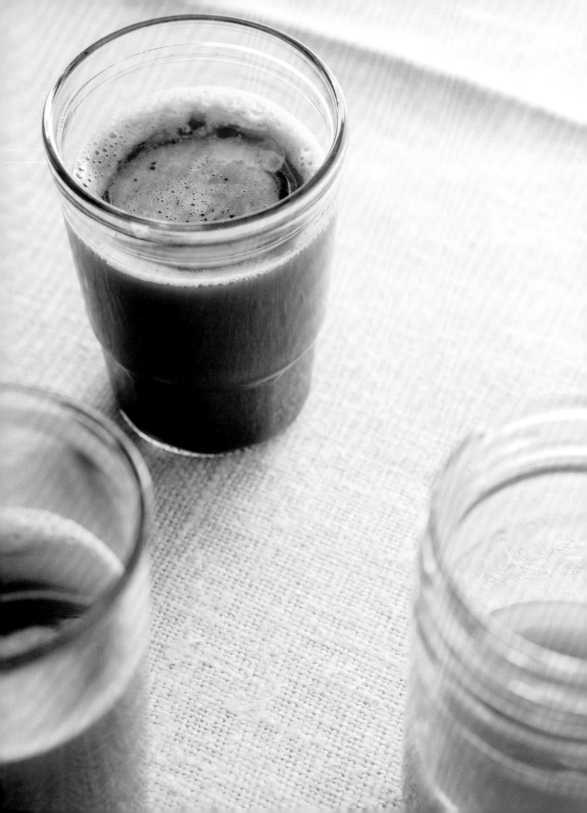

CHAPTER 12

GETTING THE MOST OUT OF YOUR CLEANSE

We talk a lot about how amazing cleansing makes us feel. Here's something to remember when you encounter your first detox headache or start crying for no reason right in the middle of an otherwise successful day: it's quite normal for cleansing to bring out some unexpected feelings in people, both physical and emotional. This chapter helps you identify some detox side effects so you don't wonder where you caught a cold or why you suddenly feel so blue.

Our cells hold on to so much, and there are a lot of negative emotions that we are storing in our bodies that we don't even think about. Anxiety and irritability can be common symptoms on a cleanse, and we urge you to let those feelings flow and ride them out. Oftentimes the release ends up feeling wonderful, just the way your physical detoxification process does.

This is all about getting back in balance, and a huge part of that is harmonizing the relationship between mind and body; toxic thoughts have a toxic effect on our bodies. We literally have the ability to make ourselves sick because toxicity in our emotions can weaken our immune system.

So please! Be gentle with yourself, especially on a cleanse. *Feel* those feelings. Cry if you need to. Own your emotions. Once you say out loud and accept what you are feeling— *I am lonely, I don't make enough money, I don't like my body, I miss my old relationship, I hate that I made that choice*—whatever it is, allow yourself to feel it. The amazing work is in doing this, because it's the hardest part. After that, letting go is often easy.

We are quite powerful and have the ability to create positive change if we are willing to go to some places that seem scary. They are really just mirrors—opportunities for us to release and move forward. Letting go of toxins—mental or physical—is a natural and in fact essential part of this process.

manage your physical symptoms

Cleansing can be an intense process, and detox symptoms are very normal. These can be emotional or physical. Remember, while your digestive system is getting a lighter load, your body is adjusting to the clean nutrients you're putting in it, and it's simultaneously ridding itself of all the junk you just don't need. A lot is going on, and sometimes that can feel a little overwhelming!

One of the most noticeable physical symptoms customers call us about is changes in digestion. Maybe your stomach is doing backflips. You're bloated. You're on the toilet too much, or not at all. Either way, something feels off. Don't worry. This is your body adjusting to this period without solid food. It may take a bit of time, but think of it as the work your system needs to do to get on track. You can help move things along by drinking 1 teaspoon of aloe vera in addition to your Aloe Vera H$_2$O (page 137).

Focus on the benefits of detoxification: more energy, regular digestion, mental clarity, clear skin, clear sinuses. There are many. But it's like anything else: it takes some hard work and a

NORMAL SYMPTOMS OF CLEANSING

- Changes in digestion
- Headaches
- Skin breakouts
- Fatigue
- Weight changes
- Trouble sleeping or changes in sleep patterns
- Irritability
- Congestion or cold symptoms

bit of a journey to get to your destination. So hang in there, and if you need support, call a friend or even our office! We are here for you.

Usually a lot of symptoms are expressed halfway through the cleanse, and many people feel the need to hibernate or take a day off from their normal routine by day 2 or 3, just because they feel their body asking for extra rest. Once you move past this, it is usually smooth sailing.

HYDRATE

Dehydration causes constipation, body acidity, and fatigue, among many other things. Continue to hydrate during your cleanse by supplementing juice intake with eight glasses of purified water per day. Water helps flush waste through the system.

REST

Rest is so crucial. The whole point of the cleanse is to allow your body to rest, and that can't happen if you are rushing around in your normal routine. Take this time as an opportunity to go to bed as early as possible and keep your schedule light.

KEEP MOVING

People ask us all the time if they are supposed to exercise on a cleanse. The truth is, just as it depends on your prior cleansing experience to understand what level you should do, the same goes for working out. We never recommend doing too much cardiovascular exercise while you are on a cleanse, as your body does need its rest. However, some light movement can improve circulation and really help get your digestive system moving and eliminating. We recommend a light walk in the morning and in the evening if possible (if you are working, try to fit it in at lunchtime; this will also distract you from all of the food being consumed by your colleagues). A gentle yoga or Pilates mat class helps many of our customers work their cores and focus on breathing without being too intense on their bodies during detoxification. This one is really up to you. We don't recommend hibernating in bed for three days straight, nor do we think you should aim to train for that marathon that is around the corner. Lie down and take it easy when you need to, and then get up and walk around the block if it is all you can do. The bottom line is that it is about balance and being gentle with yourself.

SATISFY YOUR HUNGER PANGS

Believe us, we get it—it just doesn't feel normal not to chew your food, and on top of it your stomach won't stop growling. Here is the thing: on a cleanse, your body is being nourished in a very different way than you are used to—your organs and your cells are being fed in a more direct way, and often you end up feeling oddly nourished, but with a very empty-feeling stomach. Other times, you really are just plain hungry!

We don't believe in strict rules, and we also don't believe that if you need to have a snack, the whole cleansing process is moot. However we do know that you need to snack smart, so on the next page you'll find a few suggestions for snacks if you're feeling really desperate.

VEGGIE-PEELED APPLES AND CUCUMBERS

This is such an easy trick and can be used with apples and cucumbers easily because they are simple to slice. Simply use a veggie peeler to remove the outer peel on the apple or cucumber, and then continue to use it to slice paper-thin pieces that practically melt on your tongue. You can also use the cucumbers in our Cucumber Seaweed Salad with Lemon and Sesame (at right), which we love.

CUCUMBER SEAWEED SALAD WITH LEMON AND SESAME

With delicate ribbons of cucumber, seaweed, ginger, and lemon, this Asian-inspired salad is light and refreshing with a savory bite. Just toss the ingredients together and enjoy.

SERVES 2

1 cup cucumber ribbons (see Veggie-Peeled Apples and Cucumbers, at left)

1 cup wakame seaweed, soaked for 10 minutes, then rinsed and drained

Juice of ½ lemon

1 teaspoon minced fresh ginger, peeled (optional)

Bragg Liquid Aminos

AVOCADO-CACAO-STEVIA BLENDED PUDDING

We know this might sound crazy, but avocados are one of our favorite bases for puddings and frozen dessert alternatives. Blended with the right combination of natural sweeteners and that incredible superfood, cacao, this pudding will almost make you forget about the Rocky Road sitting in the back of your freezer.

Place all of the ingredients in blender and blend until smooth. You can also freeze this if you are in the mood for ice cream. Add a pinch of cayenne for a spicy kick. And of course, if you are looking for something liquid with more substance, try making it into a smoothie or blended soup. You can't go wrong.

MAKES ABOUT 1 (6-OUNCE) SERVING

2 avocados, pitted and peeled

¼ cup raw cacao powder

2 tablespoons coconut oil

½ teaspoon powdered stevia

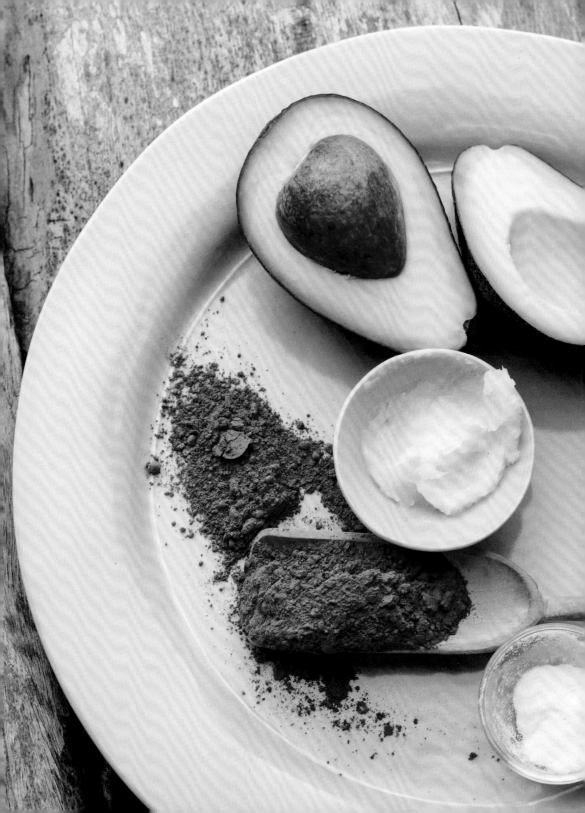

top ten ways to boost your cleanse

Cleansing is a practice that takes hard work and commitment. You're here, so you already know that. Why not maximize all of the time you've invested by boosting the power of your cleanse?

There are a few things that you can do to support all of your intention, maximize your energy, and help your body heal itself, and they all relate to self-care, a healthy lifestyle, improving digestion, maximizing elimination, and seeking relaxation—which, come to think of it, is probably why you decided to cleanse in the first place.

1. TAKE CARE OF THE BASICS The most important way to support your cleanse is by getting enough nutrition, drinking enough water, getting enough rest, and doing the right amount of movement.

2. SUPPLEMENT WITH PROBIOTICS Often when we detox, some of the good bacterial flora gets flushed out along with the bad. Taking a probiotic every day is a great way to replenish the good bacteria that your body needs to maintain a balanced state. (See the Resources, page 144, for some of our favorites.)

3. ELIMINATE WITH COLONICS It is almost counterproductive to do a cleanse if you are not moving the toxins that are being released *out* of your system. We recommend colonics or enemas as a gentle and safe way to flush out toxic waste. (For more information on colon hydrotherapy, please see the Resources, page 144.)

4. LUBRICATE WITH ALOE AND OLIVE OIL We've already talked about the benefits of Aloe Vera H_2O (page 137). Another option that can help move toxins out is to consume at least a couple of tablespoons of extra-virgin olive oil before bed to lubricate the colon and encourage elimination.

5. USE A SKIN BRUSH Skin brushing is a fantastic and cheap way to eliminate toxins. You can do this on a cleanse, but we like to incorporate it into our regular routine. It's super simple: Prior to a hot shower or bath, brush dry skin with your skin brush, starting with the soles of your feet, then your arms and legs. Go gently on your stomach and chest. Always brush upward toward your heart. Dry brushing increases circulation, sloughs off dead skin cells, opens pores, and stimulates the lymphatic system, which helps the toxins move on out. We find it reduces bloating and generally makes us feel lighter.

6. GET A MASSAGE Everybody loves a great massage! Relaxation is just what you need when you are smack in the middle of an intense detox—heck, we recommend one before, during, *and* after! But because that's not exactly possible for most people, try to incorporate at least one, or maybe a reflexology session (see opposite page), into your cleanse. You will be surprised how much emotion and stress can be released when you're lying on a massage table, and a main purpose of cleansing is to release those emotional toxins as well.

7. SCHEDULE A REFLEXOLOGY SESSION

Reflexology is a common alternative therapy that involves putting pressure on certain reflex points in the hands and feet. These pressure points correspond to different organs and parts of the body and, when utilized properly, can have a healing effect. One way that we like to use reflexology while cleansing is to focus on pressure points associated with digestion. This can help aid in elimination and get waste moving through the system. It is also great if you are experiencing uncomfortable symptoms such as headaches.

8. MEDITATE Few activities offer the grounding of a good meditation session. While it can be a transformative experience if you are familiar with the practice, it can be an intimidating prospect if you've never tried it. For beginners, we have a few simple tips to get you started on your own practice, which is mostly about quiet and being present:

- Find a relaxing, quiet place. This can be as specific as a certain corner of your favorite room. (Don't forget to turn off your phone!)

- Stretch for a few minutes before you begin. This will make you more comfortable.

- Start with the breath. Breathe in and out slowly to relax your muscles and quiet your mind. Once your mind is quiet, try to feel your body parts without thinking about them.

- Focus on your aspiration. Meditating is an active practice, and it requires full attention to a single purpose. (For instance, getting past a certain fear.) Incorporate this purpose into your breath—feel yourself breathing it in and out as if it were a tangible object.

- Feel your frustration and go with it. It is normal for people to feel their thoughts invading what is supposed to be a quiet mind. Try to move past it and keep going. Just breathe.

- Focus on your heart. Think about your open heart and how much you have to be grateful for. Naturally, your thoughts will retreat.

Be patient with yourself and practice meditation sincerely and regularly if you can, even if for just fifteen minutes at a time. If you are interested in expanding your understanding and practice, visit www.tm.org to explore Transcendental Meditation. We took a course a couple of years ago that was really amazing and gave us a greater understanding of how a meditation practice can realistically be worked into our daily lives and help us through life's difficult times.

9. SLIP INTO AN INFRARED SAUNA As you may know, the skin is the largest organ, and it is an *elimination* organ. For centuries, people have used different means to sweat out toxins through their skin, from sweat lodges to bathhouses. Infrared saunas came onto the market in more recent years and have truly restorative, detoxifying powers—we're obsessed with them. They produce immediate effects by moving the stuff you want to get rid of out of your system quickly. They also have long-term healing effects if used on a regular basis. Infrared saunas use far-infrared heat, a wavelength of light that increases the core temperature of the body and probes deeply into the layers of the skin, to relieve pain and promote weight loss. The heat penetrates to the cellular level; you will feel the difference compared to a traditional sauna. This heat opens up the blood vessels, allowing oxygen to penetrate deeply and increasing circulation. While using an infrared sauna is a great supplement to a cleanse, the cumulative effect of using one regularly is very powerful (see note below). If you can find one in your area, you will definitely notice the benefits (see the Resources, page 144).

10. DETOXIFY WITH BATH SALTS Taking a detox bath is another way to get waste moving through the body and out of the pores. Salt water is absorbed by the skin and stimulates the lymph system to get blood flowing, just like a sauna. The sulfates in the salts stimulate digestive enzymes as well and flush toxins and heavy metals from the cells (see note below).

Note: Both infrared saunas and detox salt baths can increase your heart rate. Please check with a doctor to make sure these treatments are safe for you.

easing out of your cleanse

Now that you've done this amazing work to revamp your system, we hope you can see and feel the difference in your energy level, skin quality, weight, and digestive system. Congratulations; you just accomplished something major and you deserve to celebrate! You're probably eager to reward yourself by splurging on a big meal, but unfortunately, your body isn't ready for that yet.

We recommend that you break your cleanse by consuming three small meals consisting of one solid meal and two liquid meals, the first day afterward. Keep these meals in line with the elimination diet that you followed during your precleanse. Here's a sample menu for the first and second day after a cleanse.

EASY SALT BATH SOAK

You can make this detoxifying salt soak in your own kitchen with common ingredients.

MAKES ABOUT 1 CUP

¹⁄₃ cup Epsom salts
¹⁄₃ cup gray sea salt (we use Celtic sea salt)
¹⁄₃ cup aluminum-free baking soda
A few drops of soothing essential oil (our favorites are lavender, chamomile, neroli, geranium, and jasmine)

Combine all of the ingredients in a bowl or jar. Run a hot bath and add the mixture as water runs from the faucet. Get into the bath and soak for 15 to 20 minutes. Do this once or twice a week (but no more), and drink a cool glass of water before, during, and after the bath. Take care when getting out of the tub; you may feel a bit dizzy.

DAY ONE

- **Breakfast:** Smoothie (see chapter 8)
- **Lunch:** Big Green Detox Salad (page 137)
- **Dinner:** Our Favorite Blended Soup (page 139)
- **Snacks:** 2 to 3 juices between meals

DAY TWO

- **Breakfast:** Smoothie (see chapter 8) or Painted Fruit (page 143)
- **Lunch:** Spring Green Minestrone (page 140)
- **Dinner:** Halibut in Parchment (page 142) or for something lighter, soup or a smoothie
- **Snacks:** 2 to 3 juices between meals

Listen to your body and what it needs. You may actually find that you crave more liquid meals and don't want to fill up on heavy food. Eat according to your body's natural cues. In the week following your cleanse, try to make as many of the recipes we've provided for you as possible. That way you can be sure you are staying clean.

You should be feeling really good once you finish your cleanse. At that point, it can be

easy to take your health for granted and fall back into old patterns. The beauty of juicing and cleansing is that you can always start again.

Refer back to the precleanse guidelines (see page 113) to replace processed foods and sensitivity triggers with clean and wholesome foods. It's okay if you fall off the wagon. We're all human, and sometimes—like when you're out to dinner with friends for a special occasion—you're going to indulge. Juicing, cleansing, and eating more healthfully is a lifelong process that should make you happy and improve your daily life; it's not supposed to be painful. You may feel so much better while eating this way that you'll be inspired to make this your regular way of eating.

Be patient. You probably won't change your life in three days, but this is the start of a lifestyle change. Forget unreasonable expectations; do the work and reap the benefits slowly. One green juice once won't do it—but one green juice a day can if you let it!

Everything worthwhile in life takes some work, but this work is worth it if you stick with it. You start to look forward to the work—it becomes a part of who you are. And one day you wake up and you feel different, in the best way. It is a lifelong process—always changing and evolving to adapt to *you*. The more in tune you get with your body and your health, the better you will be at understanding cues and learning to *listen*. This is a relationship that is worth nurturing—it is the basis for a life of happiness, balance, and wellness. It is a framework for optimizing your health from the inside out.

CHEW YOUR FOOD!

Once you start eating solid food again, remember that digestion begins with the simple act of chewing. Chewing initiates the release of digestive enzymes that break down food for maximum nutrient absorption.

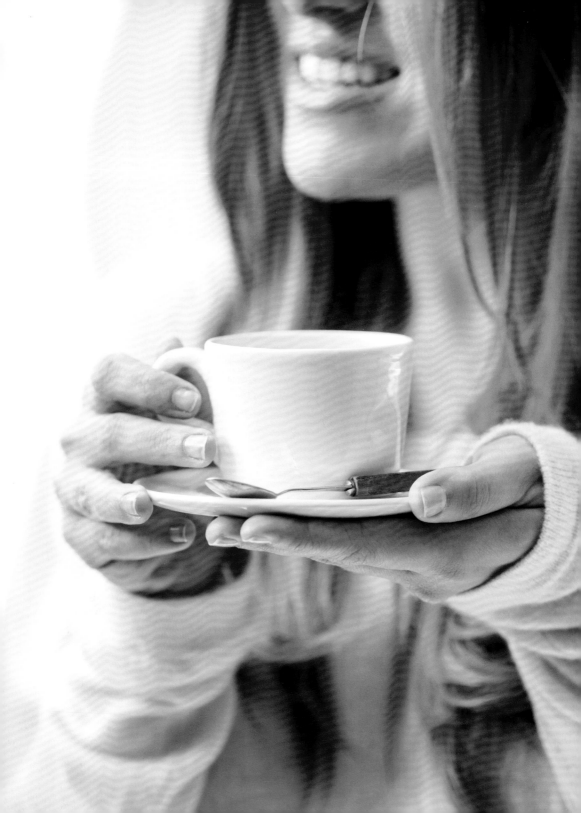

CONCLUSION

DRINK UP!

Now that we've shared our secrets with you, we hope you'll do something for us and use what you've learned. What do you want out of your day, your week, or your life? Whatever you are looking for—the stamina to finish a triathlon, the energy to chase your kids across the park, the drive to start and complete a creative project—it is all possible when you're at the top of your game. Seeking a change? Well, every change begins with one step forward.

Whoever you are and whatever you need, want, hope for, wish for, and believe, this book is for you. We are all works in progress. From the very beginning of Pressed Juicery, we have been blessed to see our customers—and now, we hope, our readers—start to crave cleaner, more nutritious foods that encourage positive choices. We have witnessed firsthand that starting your day with a green juice can retrain your palate: you really will begin to appreciate the flavors of more natural foods.

Hopefully by now you have tried a recipe or two, or at least gotten excited at the notion of changing your life in small ways (that can have huge impacts). The purpose of this book is to open the doors to healthy living, in whatever way that makes sense to you, and within a framework that is easy to follow and helps get you on the right track.

So start small, stay consistent, and don't expect huge changes overnight. This is a process, and it should never feel like a crash diet—or a crash landing. Slow and steady, people. Add green juice to your morning ritual. Have a citrus juice instead of a processed, corn syrup–filled lemonade. Drink some beets and carrots to get back to your roots, to your essence, and to everything that makes you feel grounded and balanced and good. It can seem daunting, but truly anyone can do this and you can tailor this to your needs. It can all start with just one green juice.

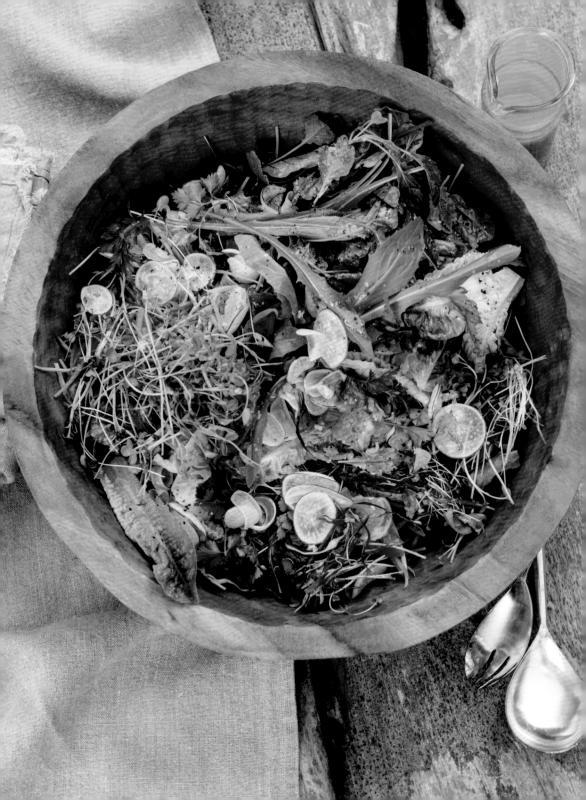

CLEANSING RECIPES

BIG GREEN DETOX SALAD

Colorful, crunchy, hydrating, and loaded with nutrition, every ingredient in this salad will help your body cleanse from the inside out. Of course it's also super delicious, and you'll love it whether you are detoxing or not.

SERVES 4 TO 6

Dressing

1 medium clove garlic, minced, or 1 small shallot, finely diced

¾ teaspoon fine sea salt

A few turns of freshly ground black pepper

1 teaspoon Dijon mustard

2½ to 3 tablespoons freshly squeezed lemon juice, to taste

½ cup extra-virgin olive oil

Salad

1 head romaine or red leaf lettuce, torn into bite-size pieces

Handful of baby kale leaves or baby Swiss chard leaves

Handful of chopped dandelion greens

Handful of fresh parsley leaves

1 cup shredded red cabbage

1 cup shredded carrot

4 radishes, julienned

Handful of sprouts (such as broccoli, radish, or clover)

Prepare the dressing: Either whisk all of the dressing ingredients together in a small bowl or place all of the ingredients in a glass jar with a lid and shake until emulsified.

Place all of the salad components in a large serving bowl. Drizzle the dressing over the salad, toss to combine, and serve immediately.

ALOE VERA H$_2$O

Aloe is very healing to the digestive tract, which is why we encourage you drink it during cleansing, but it also has other benefits, such as hydration and skin repair. You can purchase aloe vera juice in most natural food and vitamin stores—be sure to get it in the liquid and not the gel form. Combine the water and aloe vera juice and drink before bed to aid in elimination.

MAKES ABOUT 1 (8-OUNCE) SERVING

1 cup purified water

2 tablespoons aloe vera juice

CHLOROPHYLL H₂0

We have continued to mention our devotion to chlorophyll throughout these pages—and why wouldn't we? Chlorophyll is really the lifeblood of a plant, providing us with some of the most important nutrients we can get. Taken as a liquid supplement, chlorophyll can rebuild and replenish cells and soothe inflammation. Additionally, it is rich in magnesium, an alkalizing mineral that helps deliver oxygen to our tissues, bones, and muscles. You can buy chlorophyll in liquid form at most natural food and vitamin stores. Combine the water and chlorophyll and drink throughout the day for extra hydration.

MAKES 1 (8-OUNCE) SERVING

1 cup purified water
1 tablespoon liquid chlorophyll

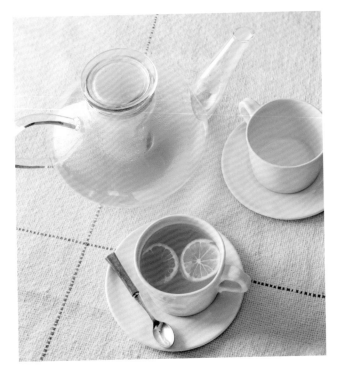

MORNING ALKALIZER

A balancing wake-up call, this is our favorite way to start the day. There is something about sipping this warm drink first thing in the morning that just feels *right*. It soothes the system and helps to balance your body's pH levels; this beverage really sets the tone for the day. We believe if you start with the Morning Alkalizer, good habits will follow. Combine all of the ingredients and drink warm like a tea.

MAKES ABOUT 1 (8-OUNCE) SERVING

1 cup warm water
1 tablespoon apple cider vinegar
1 teaspoon lemon juice
1 teaspoon manuka or raw honey

THE BEST VEGGIE BROTH

This broth is great when you are craving something savory and light—something that *tastes* like dinner, but without the heaviness of actually eating solid foods. If you want, you can save the veggies once you've strained them and snack on these as well. They will be extremely soft and much easier to digest than raw, whole pro- duce. We love to make a big pot of this broth and have it on hand for the duration of the cleanse.

MAKES ABOUT 6 CUPS

2 to 3 tablespoons extra-virgin olive oil

1 or 2 large onions, chopped, to taste

1 pound celery, chopped

1 pound carrots, chopped

1 pound leeks, white parts only, chopped

1 parsnip, chopped

Handful of any greens you have on hand

1 head broccoli, chopped into florets

4 cloves garlic

1 bay leaf

½ teaspoon black peppercorns

1 bunch fresh parsley

A few sprigs fresh thyme

Bragg Liquid Aminos (optional)

Gluten-free tamari (optional)

Heat the olive oil in a large stockpot over medium heat. As you chop your veggies, you can add them to the pot and, once you are finished, cover them with water by a couple of inches. Bring to a boil and then simmer for 1½ hours. Strain the broth through a fine sieve. You can do this a couple of times or use cheesecloth if you want to be more precise. You can add some Bragg Liquid Aminos or gluten-free tamari to the broth for more flavor.

OUR FAVORITE BLENDED SOUP

In this recipe, all you need to do is throw all of the ingre- dients in a blender, mix, and serve. The steam from the broccoli will make the soup warm but won't kill all the enzymes. You can also make a big batch of this at the beginning of your cleanse and have it for dinner each evening. Just reheat it for 2 to 3 minutes until warmed through.

MAKES ABOUT 1 (12-OUNCE) SERVING

1 zucchini, coarsely chopped

1 carrot, coarsely chopped

½ cup water

1 head broccoli, chopped into florets and lightly steamed

Pinch of cayenne pepper

½ clove garlic

Any fresh herbs you have on hand (such as a few sprigs of parsley or a pinch of thyme)

Bragg Liquid Aminos (optional; for a salty flavor)

WARM COCONUT MILLET PORRIDGE

Millet is a fantastic but underappreciated little seed that is gluten-free, alkalizing, and easy to digest. Made into a porridge, millet can be creamy and comforting. This porridge tastes a little like dulce de leche and chai tea with hints of horchata. Don't forget the toasted coconut flakes and pistachios for a special treat!

SERVES 2 TO 4

1 cup unsweetened almond milk (see chapter 7; or if you prefer to use sweetened almond milk, you can lessen the added sweetener)

¾ cup coconut milk (we use full-fat Native Forest brand)

¾ teaspoon pure vanilla extract

2 teaspoons to 1½ tablespoons raw honey, to taste (optional)

2 teaspoons to 1½ tablespoons Grade A maple syrup, to taste (optional)

⅛ teaspoon sea salt

¼ teaspoon ground cinnamon

¼ teaspoon ground cardamom

2 cups cooked millet (see Note at right)

3 tablespoons unsweetened flaked coconut

2 tablespoons chopped pistachios, almonds, or walnuts (optional)

2 tablespoons toasted unsweetened flaked coconut (optional)

In a medium saucepan, whisk together the almond milk, coconut milk, vanilla, honey, maple syrup, salt, cinnamon, and cardamom. Stir in the millet and coconut flakes, breaking up any clumps.

Bring the mixture to a boil over medium heat, then lower the heat and simmer uncovered for 10 minutes until thickened.

Remove from the heat and serve with the pistachios and toasted coconut flakes.

Note: We cook millet in a ratio of 1 part millet to 2½ parts water for about 30 minutes.

SPRING GREEN MINESTRONE

This is soup is warming, nourishing, and substantial but still feels fresh and light, just like spring. The white beans provide high-quality protein, but feel free to substitute quinoa, rice, or millet to change it up a bit. Not only is this soup easy to make, but also it cooks up very quickly.

SERVES 6

2 tablespoons extra-virgin olive oil

2 leeks, white and light green parts, thinly sliced

4 cloves garlic, thinly sliced

1 pound asparagus, trimmed and sliced on the diagonal into 1-inch pieces

1½ cups fresh or frozen green peas

2 tablespoons chopped fresh flat-leaf parsley

6 cups light chicken stock or vegetable broth, preferably homemade (see page 139)

1½ cups cooked or 1 (15-ounce) can white beans, such as cannellini or great northern, drained and rinsed

2 teaspoons sea salt (more if your stock is unsalted)

4 ounces baby spinach

In a large pot, heat the olive oil over medium heat. Add the leeks and sauté until tender, about 5 minutes. Add the garlic and sauté for another 2 minutes.

Add the asparagus, peas, and parsley and toss to coat with the oil, leeks, and garlic. Pour in the stock and stir in the white beans and sea salt. Bring to a boil, then lower the heat and simmer uncovered until the asparagus is just tender, about 5 minutes.

Stir in the spinach, taste for seasoning, and serve.

LENTIL DAL

The word *dal* really just means split pulses, or lentils. Split lentils break down to an almost creamy, mushy consistency and become soupy. Dal can be made in an infinite number of ways and is usually quite easy to digest, especially with the addition of warming spices like cumin, coriander, and turmeric.

SERVES 6

1½ tablespoons coconut oil or ghee (clarified butter)

1½ teaspoons mustard seeds

2 teaspoons ground turmeric

1½ teaspoons ground coriander

¾ teaspoon ground cumin

½ teaspoon fennel seeds

2 to 3 teaspoons sea salt, to taste

1½ cups yellow lentils

6 cups water or vegetable stock, or more as needed for thinning

Large handful of fresh cilantro, stems and leaves, chopped

Basmati rice (optional)

Melt the coconut oil in a soup pot over medium heat. Add the mustard seeds and sauté until they start to pop, about 1 minute. Add the turmeric, coriander, cumin, fennel seeds, and salt and sauté for 1 minute, or until fragrant. Add the lentils and stir to coat with the spices. Pour in the water, stir in the cilantro, and bring to a boil. Cover, lower the heat, and simmer until the lentils are soft, about 20 minutes. Taste for seasonings. Serve with basmati rice.

CAULIFLOWER TABBOULEH

Tabbouleh is typically made with bulgur wheat, but this version goes gluten-free by using grated cauliflower instead. You'll never know you're not eating a grain! Of course mineral-rich and detoxifying parsley is really the star of tabbouleh, so feel free to add lots more if you don't mind a little more chopping.

SERVES 6

1 head cauliflower, cut into florets

1 teaspoon kosher salt

2 cups diced celery, about 5 stalks

Seeds from 1 large pomegranate, about 1⅓ cups

½ cup finely diced red onion or shallot (you can soak it in ice water for 15 minutes to take the raw edge off)

½ cup extra-virgin olive oil

¼ cup chopped fresh flat-leaf parsley leaves

¼ cup fresh lemon juice

2 tablespoons chopped fresh mint leaves

¾ teaspoon ground cinnamon

¾ teaspoon ground cumin

¾ teaspoon sea salt

½ teaspoon freshly ground black pepper or to taste

Prepare a large bowl with ice water. Place the cauliflower in a large pot and cover with water by 1 inch. Add the salt. Boil for 3 to 4 minutes, until crisp-tender. Drain in a colander and immediately plunge the cauliflower in the ice water to stop the cooking.

Drain the cauliflower and transfer to a clean kitchen towel to dry a little.

Fit the grater attachment in a food processor and grate the cauliflower, or do this by hand with a box grater. It will look like barley or rice. Transfer the grated cauliflower to a serving bowl.

Stir in the remaining ingredients and toss to combine. Taste for seasonings, especially if you allow this to sit. You may need an extra pinch of salt.

HALIBUT IN PARCHMENT WITH ZUCCHINI, FENNEL, AND CAPERS

Halibut is a very mild-tasting fish and quite easy to find from wild sources, but you could also use cod for this dish. Cooking in parchment is just about the most healthful preparation for fish since steam delicately cooks it without damaging the fragile omega-3 fats. Fennel, zucchini, and lemon all work together to create a light, clean-tasting dish.

SERVES 4

2 small zucchini, very thinly sliced

1 fennel bulb, stalks trimmed away and bulb sliced as thinly as possible

8 teaspoons extra-virgin olive oil

Sea salt and freshly ground black pepper

4 (4- to 6-ounce) pieces wild halibut

2 tablespoons chopped fresh flat-leaf parsley

1 or 2 small lemons, thinly sliced into rounds

1½ tablespoons capers

Preheat the oven to 400°F. Have on hand four (12-inch-square) pieces of unbleached parchment paper.

In the center of each piece of parchment, arrange one-fourth of the zucchini and fennel slices. Drizzle 1 teaspoon of the olive oil over each vegetable mixture and sprinkle with a pinch of sea salt and a few grinds of black pepper.

Place a piece of fish on each piece of parchment, centered on top of the vegetables.

Drizzle each piece of fish with 1 teaspoon of the olive oil and season with a pinch of sea salt and a few grinds of black pepper. Sprinkle with 1½ teaspoons of parsley. Arrange 2 or 3 lemon slices on top. Sprinkle with one-fourth of the capers.

Bring two opposite sides of the parchment together and fold. Continue to fold all the way down until you reach the fish. Twist both ends of the parchment so that it looks like a hard candy wrapper. Place each packet on a baking sheet and bake for 12 to 15 minutes, depending on the thickness of the fish. Serve immediately, using caution when opening the packet.

WARM QUINOA AND VEGETABLE SALAD

Tiny seeds of warm quinoa are bouncy, fluffy, and a little nutty tasting. They're the perfect match for the crunch and colors of all the vegetables in this salad. Once you get this recipe down, you'll find ways to adapt the ingredients to fit the season.

SERVES 4 TO 6

1 cup uncooked quinoa

Sea salt

1¾ cups water

2 cups diced vegetables, such as green beans, carrots, or asparagus

2 cups chopped stemmed kale

2 scallions, thinly sliced

¼ cup diced pitted dates

⅓ cup fresh lemon juice

⅓ cup extra-virgin olive oil

Freshly ground black pepper

1 avocado, pitted, peeled, and chopped

¼ cup soaked sunflower seeds or soaked almonds, chopped

Rinse the quinoa in a bowl of water or place the quinoa in a fine-mesh sieve and rinse under cold water until the water runs clear. Transfer the quinoa to a saucepan and add a pinch of sea salt and the water. Bring to a boil, then lower the heat, cover, and simmer until the water is absorbed, about 15 minutes.

Add the vegetables, kale, scallions, and dates and cover the pot. Turn off the heat and allow to sit covered for 10 minutes.

Transfer to a serving bowl and fluff with a fork. Combine the lemon juice, olive oil, 1 teaspoon of sea salt, and freshly ground black pepper to taste in a small bowl or jar and mix well, then pour over the salad. Toss to combine. Top the salad with the avocado and sunflower seeds and serve.

PAINTED FRUIT

Painted Fruit is a creative snack or breakfast idea that we came across early on our journey on this health bandwagon. Ironically, Yogalosophy's Mandy Ingber, who made this recipe famous, was our guest editor years later on *The Chalkboard*, our online magazine. We are so thankful to her for giving us this delicious, nutritious treat, and to its original creator, Mandy's dear friend Laura Harrelson. It's really simple: you just take fresh fruit and drizzle it with this wonderful, creamy, *green* dressing. It looks a little crazy—but it's also crazy good!

SERVES 1 TO 2

1 heaping tablespoon raw almond butter

1 heaping tablespoon raw tahini

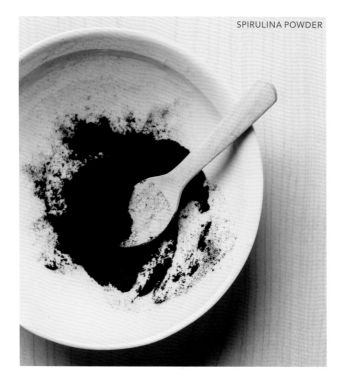

SPIRULINA POWDER

1 teaspoon agave nectar

1 tablespoon fresh lemon juice

½ teaspoon ground cinnamon, plus more for garnish

1 tablespoon hempseed or flaxseed oil

3 tablespoons spirulina powder

Freshly cut fruit (such as banana, mango, papaya, assorted berries, or a combination)

¼ teaspoon Celtic sea salt

½ cup unsweetened flaked coconut

Chopped almonds (optional)

In a small bowl, mix together the almond butter, tahini, agave nectar, lemon juice, cinnamon, and hempseed oil until creamy. Slowly stir in the spirulina powder. If the mix starts to get too thick for your liking, you may add more lemon juice and then add the remaining spirulina.

Pour or spoon the mix over the fruit. Garnish with more cinnamon, the sea salt and coconut, and almonds for added crunch. Serve immediately.

RESOURCES

colon hydrotherapists

Balance
www.balancebykamaluhia.com
Colon hydrotherapy.

The Colonic Network
www.colonic.net
Find a colonic hydrotherapist
near you.

Gentle Wellness Center
www.gentlewellnesscenter.com
Colon hydrotherapy, infrared
sauna therapy, and other wellness treatments.

Release NYC
www.releasenyc.com
Colon hydrotherapy.

SanaVita
www.sanavita.org
Center for holistic cleansing.

contributors

Kris Carr
www.crazysexylife.com
Daily motivation, inspiration,
and recipes from Kris Carr and
friends.

The Chalkboard
www.thechalkboardmag.com
Daily articles on maximizing
health and happiness.

The Honest Co.
www.honest.com
Home care products, including veggie wash.

Dr. Alejandro Junger
www.cleanprogram.com
Access to Dr. Junger's Clean
Program, which includes
supplements, community support, and recipes.

Dr. Harold Lancer
www.lancerskincare.com
Purchase Dr. Lancer's line of
skin care products and learn
about his method.

pH Miracle Living
www.phmiracleliving.com
Resources on living an alkaline
lifestyle. Organic greens supplements, books, and more.

Pressed Juicery
www.pressedjuicery.com
Information on juices, cleanses,
and other products. You can
also order our exclusive supplements and fresh, organic
coconut water.

Natalia Rose
www.detoxtheworld.com
Information on personal con-
sultations, books, and wellness
resources.

detox health centers

**Ann Wigmore Natural Health
Institute**
www.annwigmore.org
Health and wellness retreats.

Hippocrates Health Institute
www.hippocratesinst.org
Health education and healing
programs.

We Care Spa
www.wecarespa.com
Cleansing and detoxification
spa.

dining guides

Clean Plates
www.cleanplates.com
Restaurants, food news and
tips, recipes, and reviews.

Monterey Bay Aquarium
www.montereybayaquarium
.org/cr/seafoodwatch.aspx
Seafood Watch guide.

VegDining
www.vegdining.com
Online guide to vegetarian
restaurants.

equipment

Amazon
www.amazon.com
Nut milk bags, cheesecloth, and just about anything else you need.

Blendtec
www.blendtec.com
High-speed blenders.

Breville
www.breville.com
Centrifugal juicers.

Clearlight Infrared Saunas
www.infraredsauna.com
Infrared saunas for purchase.

Green Star
www.greenstar.com
Twin-gear juicers.

Hurom
www.slowjuicer.com
Masticating juicers.

Ninja
www.ninjakitchen.com
High-speed blenders.

Norwalk
www.norwalkjuicers.com
Hydraulic press juicers.

Omega
www.omegajuicers.com
Centrifugal juicers.

pH Miracle Living
www.phmiracleliving.com
Alkaline water and ionizers.

Rawsome Creations
www.rawnutmilkbag.com
Nut milk bags.

Vitamix
www.vitamix.com
High-speed blenders.

natural products and supplements

Advanced Naturals
www.advancednaturals.com
Probiotic supplements.

Billy's Infinity Greens
www.infinitygreens.com
Raw, sprouted, organic almonds and green powder supplements.

Celtic Sea Salt
www.celticseasalt.com
Our favorite source for Celtic sea salt.

Clean Program
www.cleanprogram.com
Plant-based smoothie packets.

dōTERRA
www.doterra.com
Essential oils.

E3Live
www.e3live.com
E3 algae supplement.

Larabar
www.larabar.com
Raw energy bars.

Miracle Soap
www.miraclesoap.com
Natural cleansers.

New Spirit Naturals
www.newspirit.com
Green Magic superfood bars.

Organic Creations
www.organic-creations.com
Aloe vera, liquid chlorophyll, maca powder, and vanilla beans.

Starwest Botanicals
www.starwest-botanicals.com
Liquid cayenne pepper extract.

Sunburst Superfoods
www.sunburstsuperfoods.com
Bee pollen.

Whole Foods Markets
www.wholefoodsmarket.com
Manuka honey, cacao nibs, Bragg Liquid Aminos, raw coconut sugar, oregano oil, and raw nuts and seeds.

Young Living
www.youngliving.com
Essential oils.

organic produce

LocalHarvest
www.localharvest.org
Information on community-supported agriculture.

Summerland
www.summerland.is
California-based curated produce delivery, includes recipes; national shipping available.

MEASUREMENT CONVERSIONS

VOLUME

US	Imperial	Metric
1 tablespoon	½ fl oz	15 ml
2 tablespoons	1 fl oz	30 ml
¼ cup	2 fl oz	60 ml
⅓ cup	3 fl oz	90 ml
½ cup	4 fl oz	120 ml
⅔ cup	5 fl oz (¼ pint)	150 ml
¾ cup	6 fl oz	180 ml
1 cup	8 fl oz (⅓ pint)	240 ml
1¼ cups	10 fl oz (½ pint)	300 ml
2 cups (1 pint)	16 fl oz (⅔ pint)	480 ml
2½ cups	20 fl oz (1 pint)	600 ml
1 quart	32 fl oz (1⅔ pints)	1 l

TEMPERATURE

Fahrenheit	Celsius/Gas Mark
250°F	120°C/gas mark ½
275°F	135°C/gas mark 1
300°F	150°C/gas mark 2
325°F	160°C/gas mark 3
350°F	180 or 175°C/gas mark 4
375°F	190°C/gas mark 5
400°F	200°C/gas mark 6
425°F	220°C/gas mark 7
450°F	230°C/gas mark 8
475°F	245°C/gas mark 9
500°F	260°C

LENGTH

Inch	Metric
¼ inch	6 mm
½ inch	1.25 cm
¾ inch	2 cm
1 inch	2.5 cm
6 inches (½ foot)	15 cm
12 inches (1 foot)	30 cm

WEIGHT

US/Imperial	Metric
½ oz	15 g
1 oz	30 g
2 oz	60 g
¼ lb	115 g
⅓ lb	150 g
½ lb	225 g
¾ lb	350 g
1 lb	450 g

INDEX

For Luca, Gavin, and Finley

Published in the United States by Ten Speed
Press, an imprint of the Crown Publishing Group,
a division of Random House LLC, a Penguin
Random House Company, New York.
www.crownpublishing.com
www.tenspeed.com

Ten Speed Press and the Ten Speed
Press colophon are registered trademarks
of Random House LLC.

Library of Congress Cataloging-in-Publication Data
De Castro, Carly, 1984–
    Juice: recipes for juicing, cleansing, and living
well / by Carly de Castro, Hedi Gores, and Hayden
Slater, founders of Pressed Juicery. —
First edition.
        pages cm
    Includes index.
1. Fruit juices. 2. Vegetable juices. 3. Detoxification
(Health) I. Gores, Hedi, 1976– II. Slater, Hayden,
1983– III. Title.
    TX815.D328 2014
    641.3'4—dc23
                2014000917

Hardcover ISBN: 978-1-60774-627-0
eBook ISBN: 978-1-60774-628-7

Printed in China

Design by Katy Brown
Food styling by Vivian Lui
Prop styling by Scott Horne

10 9 8 7 6 5 4 3 2 1

First Edition